Health and safety in
CARE HOMES

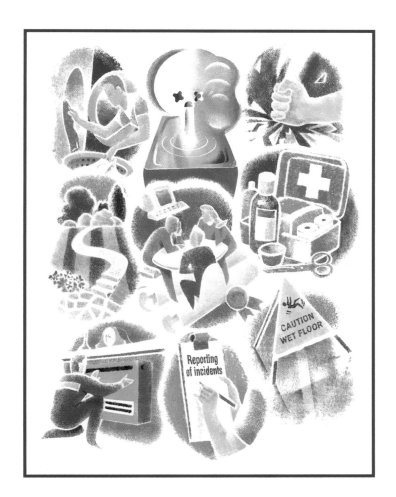

HSG220

HSE BOOKS

Contents

Continued overleaf

Health and safety in care homes

Appendices

Introduction

1   This booklet is intended for owners and managers of care homes, and for employees and safety representatives. It should help them to understand and meet their duties under health and safety legislation. It describes the main risks found in care homes, and what should be done to safeguard both workers and service users. The guidance may also be useful to other similar organisations. It has been produced by the Health and Safety Executive's Local Authority Unit, after consultation with relevant government departments and devolved administrations, local authorities, trade unions and other interested organisations.

2   The care sector caters for a wide range of needs and this guidance has tried to encompass the needs of establishments in the local authority, NHS, private and voluntary sectors. It sets out information on the responsibilities of employers and employees under health and safety legislation. The advice on implementing safe systems of work is guidance only, aimed at helping care home proprietors and others meet their health and safety obligations. Employers may of course take alternative steps to meet their duties.

3   This booklet does not include guidance on fire safety. These matters are dealt with in the booklet *Draft guide to fire precautions in existing residential care premises.*[1] It sets out basic standards for means of escape and related fire precautions. Advice on fire safety may also be obtained from the local fire prevention officer.

4   The responsibilities of care home owners are the subject of a range of legislation and regulations that are currently enforced by a number of different authorities. These include the following:
- the Health and Safety Executive (HSE), which is responsible for developing health and safety standards nationally and for the inspection and enforcement of health and safety legislation in all nursing homes, and residential care homes owned by local authorities;

- the environmental health department of the local authority, which is responsible for;
  - enforcement of health and safety legislation in private, voluntary-owned and NHS residential care homes; and
  - food safety and hygiene enforcement action in all residential care and nursing homes;
- HSE and local authorities also have responsibilities for aspects of the Working Time Regulations (see Appendix 5).

5   As of 1 April 2002, the National Care Standards Commission is responsible for the registration and inspection of all care homes in England, the Care Standards Inspectorate for Wales for care homes in Wales, and the Regulation of Care Department of the Scottish Executive for care homes in Scotland. In the light of these changes, the enforcement allocation of premises between HSE and local authorities will need to be reviewed in due course.

Occupational Health Services

6   Occupational Health Services (OHS) are concerned with the prevention of ill health in employed populations. They can help employers meet their duty of care under the HSW Act and other legislation by providing the following services:
- pre-employment assessments;
- advice on job placements;
- periodical medical examinations, including health surveillance, eg for latex allergy;
- post-sickness absence review;
- immunisations;
- health education and promotion;
- rehabilitation and return to work, eg following back injury.

7   Occupational Health Services can also help by:
- identifying work hazards that make people ill and suggesting suitable precautions;
- identifying jobs with potential for health risks;
- making first-aid arrangements; and
- providing training and education in health aspects of employment.

8   Occupational Health Services may be in-house or bought in under contract. It is important that the care home owner/manager considers the specific qualifications of occupational health personnel before employing such a service. These qualifications are as follows:

- Occupational Health Nurse - Registered General Nurse, Occupational Health Nursing Certificate/Diploma/Degree (OHNC, OHND);
- Occupational Health Physician - MB ChB or equivalent Diploma in Occupational Medicine, or Associate/Member of the Faculty of Occupational Medicine (AFOM or MFOM).

Definition of 'service user'

9   In this book, for the sake of clarity, the term 'service user' has been used to encompass people in care homes, for example patients, residents, people with learning difficulties and adults with mental health problems.

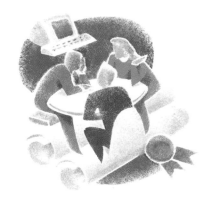

Legal framework

10   The main act relating to health and safety at work is the Health and Safety at Work etc Act 1974 (HSW Act).[2] This lays out general duties of employers, the self-employed, people in control of premises and employees.

11   The HSW Act is the umbrella legislation under which other regulations are made. These regulations usually relate to specific activities such as the management of health and safety, safety of machinery, the workplace environment, lifting and handling, control of asbestos etc.

Duties of employers to employees

12   Employers have a general duty under the HSW Act to ensure, so far as is reasonable practicable, the health, safety and welfare at work of all their employees. Under the Act, employers have to:
*   protect the health and safety of their employees;
*   protect the health and safety of others who might be affected by the way they go about their work (for example service users, volunteers, contractors and agency staff); and
*   prepare a statement of safety policy and the organisation and arrangements for carrying it out, if five or more people are employed (see Appendix 4 'Health and safety policy statements').

Duties of employees

13   Under the Act, employees have to:
*   take care of their own health and safety and that of others; and
*   co-operate with their employer.

14   If you have staff whose first language is not English, you need to make arrangements so that they can understand health and safety procedures, including training.

Duties of employers to people who are not in their employment

15   Employers, care home owners and self-employed people have responsibilities for the health and safety of people who do not work for them but may be affected by their work activities. These include service users, visitors, volunteers, and contractors' employees working on their premises. Examples of where people may be affected by the undertaking are:
*   icy pavements causing visitors to slip;
*   scalding risks to service users;
*   service users falling from windows/balconies;
*   contractors not informed of location of asbestos or a fragile roof; and
*   provision of safe equipment/substances for volunteers to use.

16   It is advisable to make enquires about contractors' procedures, including health and safety, to ascertain that they will not endanger care home employees or service users. Contact your local enforcing authority if you need to know more about the responsibilities of individuals.

Health and safety of service users

17   Care homes differ from other workplaces because they are not only a place of work but they are also a home. While meeting legal duties and providing a safe and healthy environment, they need to be maintained as pleasant places to live.

18   Service users in care homes have varying degrees of independence and therefore different needs. It is undesirable to set down strict guidelines across this range. A person living in a rehabilitation hostel will have different requirements from an elderly person in a care home. These differences need to be reflected in the design of the home, facilities and safeguards provided. Having a flexible approach should not lead to lowering of standards, but to more relevant and appropriate provision, tailored to the needs of different groups.

19   The National Health Services and Community Care Act 1990 (Community Care Act) places emphasis on promoting people's independence, treating them with dignity and respect, and encouraging them to do what they can for themselves. This may involve some level of risk-taking (known as elective risk) to enable them to develop/maintain the necessary skills associated with 'ordinary living'. A balance has to be struck to ensure the health and safety of the individual is not put at risk, and also that the independence of others is not unnecessarily restricted. However, under health and safety legislation, the home will need to protect the most vulnerable service user.

20   The key to complying with both health and safety legislation and the Community Care Act is carrying out proper risk assessments, and ensuring appropriate placements of service users according to their vulnerability and needs.

21   Employers need to ensure that they assess the vulnerability and competence of service users to judge the risk for themselves. Service users should not be exposed to the risk if they cannot make a suitable judgement. For example:
•   Is the service user mobile?
•   Can the service user manage stairs safely?
•   Can confused service users open outside doors, especially those leading to fire escape stairs?
•   Can service users go out on their own safely or must they be accompanied?
•   Can the service user bathe unsupervised?
•   Can service users judge the risk from hot water/exposed surfaces or is it necessary to control hot water and surface temperatures?

22   It is advisable to record assessments and then to review them periodically. Failure to keep such assessments up-to-date could endanger the service user and constitute a breach of legislation. There is detailed guidance on risk assessment in the 'Managing health and safety' section.

Consultation with employees

23   Good standards of health and safety cannot be achieved without the co-operation of employees. It is important for managers to work with safety representatives and employees to ensure problems are identified and resolved.

24   Two pieces of health and safety law cover consultation with employees: the Safety Representatives and Safety Committees Regulations 1977[3] deal with consulting recognised trade unions through their safety representatives; the Health and Safety (Consultation with Employees) Regulations 1996[4] cover employees who do not have trade union safety representatives. Employers must consult employees and their representatives about aspects of their health and safety at work, including:
•   any change which may substantially affect their health and safety;
•   arrangements for getting competent health and safety advice;
•   information on reducing and dealing with risks;
•   planning of health and safety training; and
•   health and safety consequences of introducing new equipment.

Health and safety law poster

25   The Health and Safety Information for Employees Regulations 1999 require that the poster *Health and safety law: What you should know*[5] is displayed in a location where employees have access. The address of the health and safety enforcing authority (ie the local environmental health department or HSE office) and the Employment Medical Advisory Service (EMAS) should be completed at the appropriate place on the poster. Alternatively, there is a leaflet with the same title which may be handed to each employee.[6]

Managing health and safety

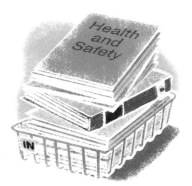

26   Good standards of health and safety in the workplace do not happen of their own accord. Safe systems of work have to be devised and implemented, staff have to be trained and equipment needs to be purchased and maintained. In other words, health and safety has to be managed as much as any other part of the business. High-performing companies recognise that managing health and safety is not only a legal duty but makes good economic sense. Employers can ill afford the losses resulting from accidents and work-related ill health. There are less obvious losses including hiring of temporary/permanent staff, lost time for management in resolving issues, higher insurance premiums, and staff training, as well as the pain and suffering of the employee(s) involved.

27   The Management of Health and Safety at Work Regulations 1999[7] apply to all work activities and require employers to manage health and safety. The Regulations and the associated Approved Code of Practice make some of the general duties of the HSW Act more specific.

The Management Regulations - key duties

Employers must:
- assess risks to staff and visitors;
- make appropriate health and safety arrangements, which must be written down if five or more people are employed;
- appoint competent persons to help them comply with health and safety law;
- establish procedures to deal with imminent danger;
- co-operate and co-ordinate with other employers and self-employed people who share the workplace; and
- provide information instruction and training.

Employees must:
- work in accordance with training and instruction given by their employer; and
- report situations which they believe to be unsafe.

28   The Regulations require health and safety to be managed by having effective health and safety arrangements (these can form part of the health and safety policy - see Appendix 4). Health and safety needs to be planned, organised, controlled, monitored and reviewed. This process will apply equally to other areas of business within the home, eg recruitment, finance, maintenance etc (see Figure 1).

29   More detailed information on managing health and safety can be found in the HSE publications *Successful health and safety management*[8] and *Managing health and safety: Five steps to success.*[9]

Risk assessment

30   The Management of Health and Safety at Work Regulations 1999 also require employers to assess the health and safety risks to both employees and others affected by the business. You should concentrate on the significant risks, not on minor ones. The assessment needs to be suitable and sufficient, not perfect.

31   A risk assessment involves carrying out a careful examination of what could cause harm to people and considering whether you have done enough to prevent harm, or whether more action needs to be taken. The aim is to make sure that no one is hurt or becomes ill from your work activities.

Definitions
Hazard: anything that can cause harm, eg chemicals, electricity, moving and handling service users.
Risk: the chance, high or low, that somebody will be harmed by the hazard.

Figure 1 Model for managing health and safety

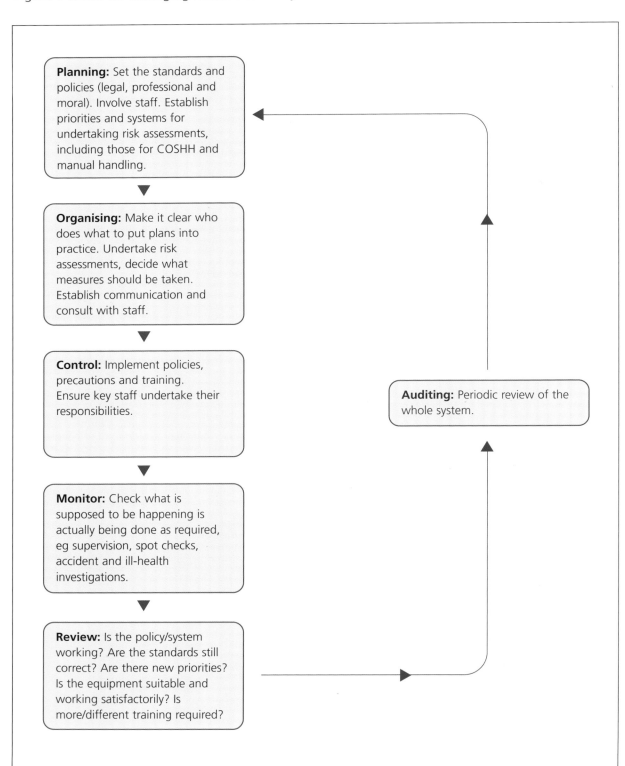

Planning: Set the standards and policies (legal, professional and moral). Involve staff. Establish priorities and systems for undertaking risk assessments, including those for COSHH and manual handling.

Organising: Make it clear who does what to put plans into practice. Undertake risk assessments, decide what measures should be taken. Establish communication and consult with staff.

Control: Implement policies, precautions and training. Ensure key staff undertake their responsibilities.

Monitor: Check what is supposed to be happening is actually being done as required, eg supervision, spot checks, accident and ill-health investigations.

Review: Is the policy/system working? Are the standards still correct? Are there new priorities? Is the equipment suitable and working satisfactorily? Is more/different training required?

Auditing: Periodic review of the whole system.

32   Some assessments may be simple and arise directly from observation, such as obstructions in the corridor creating a tripping hazard, others may be more complex, for example whether service users can go out of the home by themselves. The assessment should cover the following five steps.

Step 1 Identify the significant hazards

33   Walk around your workplace and look at the things that can cause serious harm or affect several people. It can be the physical environment, equipment, tasks or people's behaviour. Ask your employees or their representatives for their views. Accident and ill-health records can help identify hazards, as can manufacturer's instructions.

Step 2 Decide who might be harmed

34   Take into account employees including new staff, young workers, cleaners, maintenance staff, contractors, service users, visitors etc.

Step 3 Evaluate the risks and decide whether existing precautions are adequate or more should be done

35   Your aim is to make all risks small. If the risk remains high or medium, then you need to do more. Give priority to the risks that remain high or affect most people. First consider if you can get rid of the hazard altogether. For example, replace very hot radiators (above 43°C) with cool-walled ones (low-surface-temperature heat-emitters). If you cannot remove the hazard, you need to control the risk by taking additional precautions. You will need to apply the following principles, preferably in the order they are listed:

- try a less risky option, eg replace radiators next to beds and chairs as a priority;
- prevent access to the hazard, eg cover existing radiators with guards;
- organise work to reduce exposure to the hazard, eg share moving and handling tasks among staff and throughout the day;
- issue personal protective clothing, eg latex-free gloves;
- provide welfare facilities, eg washing facilities to remove contamination; and
- provide first-aid facilities.

36   Once you have identified the measures to avoid or control the risks in your assessments, they need to be implemented. Not all precautions need to be expensive and some can just be a change of working practice. You need to check that these new and existing precautions are used and continue to be effective.

Step 4 Record your findings

37   If you have five or more employees then you need to record the significant findings (hazards and conclusions) of your risk assessments and tell your staff about them. An example of a significant finding might be 'upper-floor windows restricted and checked every month'.

Step 5 Review your assessment and revise it if necessary

38   It is useful to keep records to demonstrate that you have considered all the necessary aspects. They are also useful as a reference point for when the assessments need to be reviewed (whenever circumstances change or periodically to ensure that they remain current).

39   The HSE leaflet *Five steps to risk assessment*[10] gives more details on how to assess risks in the workplace. The following examples of risk assessments show how they can be used in a care home environment.

Risk assessment: Example 1

The time periods given in the following table are purely to support the example provided.

Hazard	Who might be harmed and how	Precautions in place already	Additional precautions required and who to organise and by when	Assessment review date and by whom
Lifting heavy, bulky containers of laundry and dishwasher detergents from stores to dispensing position, **bending** under worktop (for the dishwasher) and **squeezing** behind washing machines (in the laundry)	Two kitchen staff - frequently lifting container from store to position under worktop One member of laundry staff - frequently lifting container from stores to narrow position behind washing machines One handyman - infrequent lifting for kitchen and laundry staff Medium risk of back, neck, shoulder injury	Sack trolley for moving containers Moving and handling training every 3 years for ancillary staff	Investigate the possibility and cost of using smaller containers for kitchen and laundry - chef to have done this by 2 weeks' time Make a low movable platform for the container to sit on under the worktop so the container can be slid in and out of position - handyman to make by next month Make a low movable platform for the container to sit behind washing machines' worktops so the container can be slid in and out of position - handyman to make by next month When replacing machines ensure detergent position sited better	Home manager to check additional precautions being used in 8 weeks' time Home manager to review effectiveness of moving and handling training by next month and organise refresher training Low risk if all precautions used

Risk assessment: Example 2

Hazard

Bedrails (cot sides)

Who might be harmed and how

Potential for service users to be injured or asphyxiated from entanglement with bedrails

Service users may be injured climbing over bedrails

Service users may be injured falling out of bed if bedrails not used

Precautions

Detailed assessment of service user's needs and capabilities including:

* Can tucked in sheets/blankets be used instead of bedrails?
* Can any necessary body positioning device be used instead?
* Can a height-adjustable bed be used?
* Can something be placed on the floor to cushion a fall?
* Can an alarm system be used to alert staff that someone has moved from their normal position?
* Can the mattress be placed on the floor (for high-risk service users and in exceptional circumstances)?

If bedrails are to be used, then check that they:

* are compatible with the type of bed;
* are compatible with the service user;
* are fitted to the bed correctly to prevent entrapment. There should be no gaps, for example, between the lower bar of the bedrail and the top of the mattress, or between the mattress, the end of the bedrail and the headboard or wall. The mattress should not compress easily along its edge. In some cases, a cot bumper can be used to close any hazardous gaps;
* are maintained in working order; and
* have properly engaged locking mechanisms and staff are trained to use these correctly.

Further advice on the safe use of bedrails is available from the Medical Devices Agency (see the 'Further information' section for the address).

Contact manufacturers for advice on compatibility with bed, fitting and maintenance of bedrails.

Findings

If the above factors are in place, then the risk to service users is low. Record assessment of need for bedrails, type of bedrail to be used with type of bed, action taken to minimise gaps, maintenance etc.

Review

Care staff to check bedrail position and working order frequently, eg daily.

Key worker to regularly review the need for bedrails. A new risk assessment will need to be carried out if the bed, mattress or bedrail change or the service user's needs change.

It is advisable to obtain consent before using bedrails.

Health and safety assistance

40   You are required to appoint one or more 'competent persons' to assist you in complying with health and safety law. You must ensure that these people have enough time and resources to fulfil their responsibilities.

41   A competent person is someone who has sufficient training and experience or knowledge (an understanding of relevant statutory requirements and an appreciation of the hazards involved) to do the required job.

Training

42   You must make sure that employees have suitable information, instruction and training in order to do the job safely. Training is an important way of achieving health and safety compliance and helps to convert information into safe working practices. All employees, including management, need to be appropriately trained but particular attention needs to be paid to:

* the induction and training of new workers, young workers, part-time and nightshift workers;
* those given specific responsibilities in the health and safety policy;
* employees who transfer, take on new

responsibilities or deputise, or staff who return to work after extended absence; and

- changes in equipment and systems of work or procedures.

43   The risk assessment should identify where specific training is required, such as dealing with aggressive people. The competence of staff should be monitored. Refresher or update training may be needed to ensure that staff maintain their skills.

Training checklist

The following checklist shows what may need to be considered when preparing a typical training programme.

Decide what training is required and who needs it

What area of knowledge/skills needs improvement, eg moving and handling, clinical waste procedures etc?

How is the trainee to be selected? Consult safety representatives and staff.

Selection should take account of the physical and mental demands of the job.

Staff may need to be selected into priority order. How much does the trainee already know about safe working practices?

Decide what the objectives are

What should the training achieve?

Prepare a list of all the points training should cover, for example:

- relevant law, policies and procedures;
- what equipment or substance to use;
- how the equipment or substance works and what it does;
- what dangers are associated with its use, including accidental spillage, ill health;
- what safety precautions are needed and how they protect the user;
- how to clean equipment safely;
- maintenance of equipment;
- what to do if equipment seems faulty;
- what personal protective equipment to wear.

Choose the method of training

Will training be 'on' or 'off' the job?
Who will carry out the training?
Who will supervise the training?
What records will be kept?

Carry out the training

Choose someone or an organisation who can deliver the training effectively.

If training is on the job, set the trainee to work under close supervision and make sure the supervisor has the time and knowledge to supervise effectively.

Make sure the supervisor watches to see that dangerous practices do not develop.

Check the training has worked

Check that the trainee understood the training, eg by the end of course organise quizzes, questionnaires, tests. Does the trainee know how to carry out the work properly and safely? This can be checked by working alongside a supervisor immediately post-course and ideally sometime later.

Make the sure trainee can be left to work safely without close supervision and monitor performance on a regular basis. (It should be noted that as relationships strengthen between staff and service users, the staff may be encouraged to undertake unsafe tasks by service users requiring a favour.)

Periodically review the effectiveness of the training provided.

Young workers

44   The Management of Health and Safety at Work Regulations 1999 particularly require that young persons (those under 18) should not be employed unless there has been a specific risk assessment for them, taking into account:

- inexperience, lack of awareness of risks and immaturity of young people;
- the workplace and equipment;
- the nature and degree of exposure to harm;
- organisation of processes and activities; and
- training.

More detailed information can be found in the HSE publication *Young people at work* (see 'Further reading').

Reporting of incidents

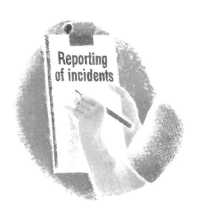

45   The Reporting of Injuries, Diseases and Dangerous Occurrences Regulations 1995 (RIDDOR) require employers and others to report certain types of injury, occupational ill health and dangerous occurrences that arise out of or in connection with work.

How and when to report an incident

46   Reporting an incident does not suggest in any way that you accept responsibility for the event or that an offence has been committed; it is simply informing the enforcing authority that an incident has occurred at your premises. Failure to report a reportable injury, dangerous occurrence or disease described in RIDDOR within the set time (see next paragraph) is a criminal offence and may result in prosecution.

47   You must report fatal accidents, accidents resulting in major injuries, accidents to people who are not at work and dangerous occurrences to the Incident Contact Centre (ICC) at the following address without delay:
Incident Contact Centre
Caerphilly Business Park
Caerphilly
CF83 3GG
Telephone: 0845 300 9923
Fax: 0845 300 9924
www.riddor.gov.uk

48   You must report other accidents in writing on the relevant form (Form F2508) within ten days - see Appendix 2. Diseases must be notified in writing (on Form F2508A) as soon as possible - see Appendix 3.

49   The following paragraphs give a summary of the requirements, but are by no means a comprehensive or exhaustive statement of law. The full text of the Regulations and relevant guidance are available in *A guide to the Reporting of Injuries, Diseases and Dangerous Occurrences Regulations 1995*[11] and there is further guidance in *The Reporting of Injuries, Diseases and Dangerous Occurrences Regulations 1995: Guide for employers in the healthcare sector.*[12]

What needs to be reported?

50   Under RIDDOR, some work-related accidents, diseases and dangerous occurrences must be reported.

51   The following are reportable if they arise 'out of or in connection with work':
- accidents that result in an employee or a self-employed person dying, suffering a major injury, or being absent from work or unable to do their normal duties for more than three days;
- accidents that result in a person not at work suffering an injury and being taken to a hospital;
- an employee or self-employed person suffering one of the specified work-related diseases; or
- one of the specified 'dangerous occurrences' - these do not necessarily result in injury but have the potential to do significant harm.

52   'Accidents' include acts of physical violence to people at work, but not violence to others such as service users or visitors.

53   You do not need to report accidents arising directly from the conduct of an operation, examination or other medical treatment carried out or supervised by a doctor or dentist. Professional misconduct can be reported to the General Medical Council (GMC) for doctors and the United Kingdom Central Council (UKCC) for nurses.

Who should report?

54   Employers, the self-employed and those in control of work premises have duties under the Regulations. The duty to notify and report rests with the 'responsible person'. This may be the employer of an injured person, a self-employed person, or someone in control of premises where work is carried out. Who the responsible person is depends on the circumstances of the notifiable event, as shown in Table 1.

Table 1 Responsible persons

Reportable event	Injured person	Responsible person
Death, major injury, over-3-day injury or case of disease	Employee at work	Employer
Death, major injury or over-3-day injury	Self-employed person at work in premises controlled by someone else	Person in control of the premises
Major injury, over-3-day injury or case of disease	Self-employed person on their own premises	Self-employed person or someone acting on their behalf
Death or reportable injury	A person not at work	Person in control of the premises
Dangerous occurrence		Person in control of the premises

Table 2 Examples of accidents to service users

Reportable	Not reportable
A confused service user falls from a window on an upper floor and is badly injured and taken to hospital	A frail, elderly person, not identified as requiring special supervision, falls and is taken to hospital. There are no obstructions or defects in the premises that contributed to the fall
A service user is scalded by hot bath water and is taken to hospital	A service user is attacked by another service user and taken to hospital as a result of the injuries sustained
A service user falls out of bed and is taken to hospital. Assessment had identified the need for bedrails but they had not been fitted	A service user falls out of bed and is taken to hospital. There was a detailed assessment in the care plan that bedrails were not appropriate

Table 3 Examples of diseases

Reportable	Non reportable
A nurse contracts TB after nursing a service user with TB	A care assistant becomes colonised with MRSA
A secretary suffers from a work-related upper limb disorder	A carer catches scabies, probably from a service user (infestation so not reportable)
A care assistant suffers dermatitis associated with wearing latex gloves during service user care	A member of staff has dermatitis caused by factors not related to work
A member of staff suffers from asthma after using glutaraldehyde	A nurse catches flu, which is widespread in the local community

Table 4 Examples of dangerous occurrences

Reportable	Not reportable
A person hoist fails due to overload	A domestic suffers a needlestick injury, the source of the sharp is unknown
Asbestos is released from ducting during maintenance work	A urine specimen container is broken and the contents are spilled
A fire is caused by a short circuit in a heater	Contractors cause a short circuit but it does not lead to a fire or explosion
A nurse has a needlestick injury with a needle that has been used on someone with a blood-borne virus	A nurse is injured by a needle that has not been in contact with a service user

Record-keeping

55   You must keep a record of any reportable injury, diseases or dangerous occurrence for three years from the date of the incident. This must include:
- the name and occupation of employee affected;
- the name and status (eg service user, visitor) of non-employee affected;
- a brief description of the circumstances; and
- the date and method of report to enforcing authority.

56   The employer should also keep a record of any reportable disease. These records should include:
- the date of diagnosis of the disease;
- the name and occupation of the person affected;
- the name or nature of the disease; and
- the date and method of report to enforcing authority.

57   You can keep the record in any form you wish, for example by keeping copies of completed report forms in a file or recording the details on a computer. It is good practice to record other accidents and near-misses as you can used the data collected from incidents to improve your health and safety performance.

Table 5 Reportability of accidents

Person involved	Accident details	Type of injury	Reportable under RIDDOR
Employee	Fell off step ladder while cleaning cupboard in care home. Sustained broken arm	Major injury	Contact Incident Contact Centre (ICC)
Employee	Hurt back while lifting service user out of bath. Off work for 5 days	Over-3-day injury	Send F2508 within 10 days to ICC
Employee	Hurt back while digging garden at home (employee's home). Off work for 5 days		Not reportable. Accident not at work
Employee	Banged head on door at work. Taken to hospital. Detained for 24 hours. Returned to work next day	Major injury	Contact ICC
Service user	Tripped over vacuum cleaner and broke leg	Major injury	Contact ICC
Service user	Died in sleep		Not reportable if natural causes
Employee driver	Twisted ankle while assisting service user out of vehicle. Unable to drive for 4 days but assists in home with light duties	Over 3-day injury	Send F2508 within 10 days to ICC
Employee	Cut finger while preparing food for service users. No time taken off work		Not reportable as not away from work for more than 3 days
Part-time employee	Normally works Mon-Wed. Injured back while lifting service user on Monday. Absent Tuesday and Wednesday. On return to work the following Monday reports that injury did not abate until Friday	Over-3-day injury	Send F2508 within 10 days to ICC
Visitor	Tripped over frayed carpet. Taken to hospital	Injury to member of public	Contact ICC
Employee	Bitten by a service user. Off work for 4 days	Over-3-day injury	Send F2508 to ICC within 10 days

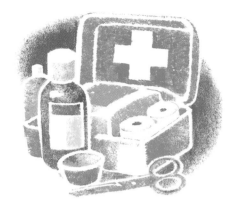

First aid

58   Under the Health and Safety (First-Aid) Regulations 1981, workplaces should have first-aid provision. The extent it should take depends on various factors, including the nature and degree of the hazards at work, whether there is shift working, what medical services are available, and the number of employees. The HSE book *First aid at work*[13] contains an Approved Code of Practice and guidance to help employers meet their obligations.

59   The minimum requirement for any workplace is that when people are at work (including nightshifts), there should be at least one appointed person who will take charge in an emergency situation. This includes being responsible for calling an ambulance and looking after the first-aid equipment, for example restocking the first-aid box. An appointed person should be available at all times while people are working on-site; this may mean appointing more than one. It is recommended that an appointed person should have received emergency first-aid training.

60   Although the Regulations only refer to facilities for employees, it is recommended that you extend these to cover service users and visitors. You may wish to consider providing qualified first-aiders. They can fulfil the duties of an appointed person. A first-aider is someone who has undergone a training course in administering first aid at work and holds a current first aid at work certificate. The training course must be approved by HSE - contact the First Aid Approvals Office (Tel: 0161 952 8322). First-aiders should receive refresher training every three years.

61   There are no hard and fast rules on the number of appointed persons/first-aiders you should have, it depends on the circumstances of your business. Table 6 suggests some numbers but consideration should also be given to shift work.

Table 6 Suggested numbers of first-aid personnel

Category of risk	Numbers employed at any location	Suggested number of first-aid personnel
Lower risk, eg shops, offices, libraries	Fewer than 50	At least one appointed person
	50-100	At least one first-aider
Medium risk, eg warehousing, most care homes	Fewer than 50	At least one appointed person
	20-100	At least one first-aider for up to every 50 employed

62   A first-aid box should be provided and should contain only items that a first-aider has been trained to use. It should not contain medication of any kind. It should be kept adequately stocked. Where there is a risk of infection then disposable latex-free gloves should be provided (see 'Latex sensitisation' section).

63   All cases dealt with should be recorded by the first-aider or appointed person. Records should include at least the name of the casualty, date, time and circumstances of the accident, with details of the injury sustained and any treatment given. Employees or their representatives may wish to inspect these records so they should be available for them to do so.

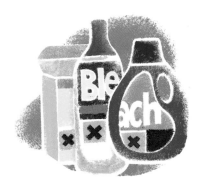

Hazardous substances

64   The Control of Substances Hazardous to Health Regulations 1999 (COSHH)[14] require employers to prevent or control exposure to hazardous substances (including chemicals, dust, fumes, micro-organisms) at work. This duty applies to employees, service users, visitors etc.

COSHH - key duties

Employers must:
- assess the risk to their employees and others from exposure to hazardous substances at work;
- introduce appropriate precautions to prevent or control the risk that has been identified;
- ensure that the precautions are used, equipment is properly maintained and procedures are followed;
- where necessary, monitor the exposure of the employees and undertake health surveillance; and
- inform, instruct and train employees about the risks and precautions to be taken.

65   Hazardous substances used in care homes include some cleaning materials, disinfectants and micro-organisms (associated with clinical waste or soiled laundry).

66   Employers must assess the health risk faced by their employees, service users and visitors, and decide on the action they need to take to prevent or control exposure to hazardous substances. The results of the assessment should be made known to the employees or their representative.

COSHH assessment

67   When undertaking a COSHH assessment, employers should look at the work activities and ask the following questions:
- What substances are present and in what form?
- What harmful effects are possible?
- Where and how are the substances stored, used and handled?
- Are harmful fumes produced, especially if products are mixed?
- Can a safer substance be used?
- Who could be affected, to what extent, for how long and under what circumstances?
- How likely is it that exposure will happen?
- Are precautions required, such as ventilation and protective equipment?

68   Certain information about products may be found on labels, which on hazardous substances may include risk phrases such as 'avoid contact with skin'. If the information is not readily available on the label or an advisory leaflet, then a data sheet for that product should be obtained from the supplier or manufacturer. They have a legal duty to supply such information.

69   COSHH assessments should be relatively simple in a care home. First of all you need to establish what products and biological hazards (eg clinical waste or soiled laundry) are in the home. Identify if any less harmful products can be used to decrease the risk. If products cannot be replaced, then you need to reduce the potential for exposure to your staff and service users. This means that you will need to provide staff with precautions such as good ventilation and protective equipment.

70   Protective equipment should only be used if it is not reasonably practicable to provide other precautions. Toilet cleaners and polishes may only require the use of rubber gloves, whereas descalers and oven cleaners may require heavy-duty gloves, goggles or face shields and a well ventilated area while the products are being used. Many of the risks for the hazardous substances in a care home are the same so you can group similar chemicals or hazards together and undertake a single generic assessment.

71   It is extremely important that staff are given information, instruction and training on how to use the product safely, how to clear up spillages, and how to check and wear protective equipment, eg goggles, face shields, gloves etc. If items of equipment are faulty, they should be replaced or repaired.

72   All cleaning materials should be kept out of reach of vulnerable service users, for example locked in a cupboard when not in use. There have been deaths in the past where service users in care homes have mistaken cleaning fluids for a drink. In many cases, the fluid had been decanted into an unmarked container.

Tips

Some chemicals that are relatively harmless on their own may become extremely hazardous when mixed, for example toilet cleaner and bleach may react together to give off chlorine gas. It is important that the employees are made aware of the potential hazards.

Where health and safety information is contained on the label, the contents should not be decanted into smaller containers unless fully labelled in line with the original bottle.

Drugs and medicines

73   Drugs and medicines can be dangerous if misused. Some may also require care when handled and administered as they can cause health hazards to staff, eg Ipecacuana, antibiotic powders, cytotoxic drugs etc. Other drugs require specific storage conditions. Advice may be obtained from pharmacists.

74   All drugs should be correctly labelled and procedures should be adopted to ensure safe administration either by service users or by staff who have received appropriate training. Drugs should be kept in secure location to prevent misuse and unauthorised access.

Latex sensitisation

75   Most medical gloves are made from natural latex rubber. It is a durable, flexible material that affords a high degree of protection from many micro-organisms. It is also used in a range of medical devices. As the use of such products has increased, latex allergy and sensitisation has been identified as a problem. This is particularly so among those in the care sector where increased use of gloves has occurred. Latex exposure can lead to irritation and allergic reactions. See the HSE leaflet *Latex and you*[15] for more details.

76   There are a number of different types of latex glove available. All of these present a particular risk of

skin sensitisation, but the risk is reduced in gloves with lower levels of latex protein and processed chemicals. Powdered gloves increase the risk of respiratory sensitisation and should not be used.

77   Latex falls under the Control of Substances Hazardous to Health Regulations 1999 (COSHH) and therefore you must either prevent or control the risk of latex sensitisation. In practice, the protective measures likely to be identified by a suitable and sufficient assessment may include one or more of the following:
- implementing a general policy on latex use including:
  - the risk of exposure to latex;
  - when and when not to use latex gloves;
  - arrangements for health checks/surveillance;
  - help in recognising the symptoms of sensitisation;
  - the action needed if staff are affected by latex;
- limiting exposure by not wearing gloves when there is no risk of infection, eg when making beds (if not wet/soiled), or when other types of gloves are more appropriate, eg for washing up;
- ensuring that where gloves have to be worn as protective equipment, latex-free gloves are available;
- implementing a glove purchasing policy which specifies latex-free or low levels of latex protein;
- washing hands after removing gloves. Barrier creams should not be used in conjunction with latex gloves as they may increase the penetration of allergens;
- implementing a health surveillance programme including pre-employment screening for employees exposed to latex;
- ensuring the latex policy covers the action needed to protect staff who are sensitised to latex. This may include providing them with gloves made of an alternative material to latex and reviewing the risks to their health from contact with other latex products;
- ensuring that the policy on latex is brought to the attention of all employees.

78   If staff develop symptoms that may be caused from exposure to latex, you should refer them to your occupational health practitioner or their GP.

Control of infection

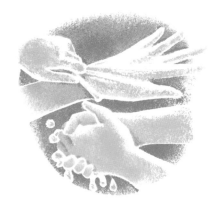

79   Control of infection is an important consideration throughout the care home environment. There may be the potential for exposure to a range of human pathogens with the consequent risk of harm or disease. All homes should have an infection control policy that addresses such issues as:

- education and training of staff in infection control issues;
- protocols on handwashing;
- service user isolation;
- aseptic procedures;
- disinfection and decontamination including domestic cleaning;
- ill-health reporting and recording;
- monitoring, surveillance and audit;
- prevention of exposure to blood-borne viruses, including prevention of sharps injuries and immunisation policies for at risk staff;
- use of personal protective equipment including powder-free latex gloves;
- generation, collection and disposal of clinical waste.

Clinical waste

80   Staff employed in care homes may have to deal with body fluids and wastes (termed clinical waste) that are potentially hazardous to the handler. Clinical waste is covered by a number of pieces of legislation including the Control of Substances Hazardous to Health Regulations 1999 (COSHH) - see 'Hazardous substances' section.

81   Clinical waste is divided into five categories, see Table 7. The category determines the necessary packaging and labelling requirements. If a risk assessment shows that sanitary towels, tampons, nappies, stoma bags, incontinence pads and other similar wastes (providing they do not contain sharps), do not present a significant risk of infection, they need not be classified as clinical waste. However, the offensiveness of non-infectious waste needs to be taken into account when deciding how to package waste for disposal.

Table 7 Types of clinical waste

Waste group	Type of clinical waste
Group A	Identifiable human tissue, blood, soiled surgical dressings, swabs and other similar soiled waste. Other waste materials, eg from infection disease cases, excluding any in Groups B-E.
Group B	Discarded syringe needles, cartridges, broken glass and any other contaminated disposable sharp instruments or items.
Group C	Microbiological cultures and potentially infected waste from pathology departments and other clinical or research laboratories
Group D	Drugs or other pharmaceutical products
Group E	Items used to dispose of urine, faeces and other bodily secretions or excretions that do not fall within Group A. This includes the use of disposable bedpans or bedpan liners, incontinence pads, stoma bags and urine containers*

* Where the risk assessment shows there is no infection risk, Group E waste is not clinical waste as defined.

82   There should be suitable procedures for handling clinical waste. You need to consider:

- training and information;
- personal hygiene;
- personal protective equipment;
- immunisation;
- segregation;
- handling;
- packaging;
- labelling;
- storage;
- transport on-site and off-site;
- accidents/incidents and spillages; and
- treatment and disposal.

83   Staff should be given clear information, instruction and training on deciding what is clinical waste and what constitutes domestic waste. There is a widely used system of colour-coding to aid the process of waste segregation:

- Yellow - Group A clinical waste for incineration or other suitable means of disposal
- Yellow with black stripes - non-infectious waste, eg Group E and sanpro (sanitary towels, tampons, nappies, stoma bags, incontinence pads). Waste suitable for landfill or other means of disposal
- Black - non-clinical or household waste

84   Disposable plastic coloured sacks should only be fixed three-quarters full and then sealed-off by tying the neck. As of January 2002, if clinical waste is to be taken off-site then it has to be transported in suitable UN type approved rigid packaging.

85   Group B waste should be disposed of in sharps containers which meet the requirements of BS 7320: 1990 and are UN type approved. When the bin is three-quarters full the containers should be sealed. Sharps containers should not be placed in bags prior to disposal. Sharps containers should not be left lying around where children and other vulnerable people could gain access. There have been a number of incidents where children have received needlestick injuries from 'playing' with sharps boxes.

86   Some sharps may be hazardous in other ways. For example, they may be contaminated with cytotoxic drugs or other potentially harmful pharmaceuticals. The use of sharps boxes, UN type approved for UN3291 waste, will still give adequate protection in these circumstances. It should be remembered that such waste is also likely to be special waste and you should contact your waste authority for more details. Broken glass should also be put into sharps containers.

87   Needles should not be resheathed after use but put directly into the sharps bin. Used needles should not be disposed of in domestic waste or in soft drink cans, plastic bottles or similar containers.

Storage
88   Clinical waste containers may need to be stored before removal from the home. They should not be allowed to accumulate in corridors or other places accessible to members of the public. The area where the waste is stored should be:

- designated for clinical waste only;
- enclosed and secure.

Training
89   All employees who are required to handle and move clinical waste should be adequately trained in safe procedures and how to deal with spillages or other incidents. Refresher training will also be required from time to time. It is also advisable to keep training records.

Accidents and incidents
90   Care home owners/managers should identify procedures for dealing with accidents and incidents involving clinical waste including spillages. Staff need to be fully aware of the procedures.

91   Procedures will need to be drawn up to cover arrangements for suitable medical advice and counselling if sharps injuries occur.

92   Spillage kits containing disposable aprons, latex-free gloves, clinical waste bag and tag, paper towels, sodium hypochlorite and instructions help to ensure staff take the correct action.

Disposal of waste
93   Safe disposal of clinical waste is the responsibility of the care home owner. Transfer notes or other documentation help to establish that clinical waste has been disposed of correctly. The domestic waste collection service should not be used for clinical waste. More detailed information can be found in the HSE book *Safe disposal of clinical waste.*[16]

Risks from blood and body fluids
94   Healthcare workers are sometimes at risk from infections carried in blood and body fluids, for example hepatitis B. Some staff in care homes may also face the same risk.

95   As there is a risk of acquiring such an infection due to work activity, the employer/owner should undertake a COSHH assessment (see 'Hazardous substances' section). In practice, such assessments are often linked to the infection control policy and needlestick injuries policy.

96   Steps can be taken to minimise the risk of contamination from infected blood/body fluids. Precautions include:

- covering cuts/grazes with waterproof dressings before commencing work;
- good personal hygiene standards - thorough handwashing after contact with blood and body fluids;
- good environmental hygiene - cleaning and disinfecting contaminated equipment (if not disposable) after use and keeping the environment clean;
- wearing latex-free gloves, disposable aprons etc for high-risk/messy activities (see 'Latex sensitisation' section).

97   Staff should have clear instructions on how to clear up and disinfect a spillage of infected blood/body fluids. This should include how to mop up the spillage, preparing the chemicals, applying the chemicals to the spillage site and the final clearing up. In addition, you should specify the safety measures that staff should take such as how much ventilation is required and what personal protective equipment should be worn. It is often useful to have such a procedure written down and kept with the spillage kit/chemicals for disinfecting blood/body fluid spills.

98   In homes where there is known to be a high incidence of hepatitis B among service users, employers should offer staff appropriate immunisation. Employers should have an agreed arrangement with an occupational health service (see the Introduction to this book) or a GP for the immunisation of staff. Once staff have been immunised, there will need to be periodic checks to ensure that they remain adequately protected by the vaccine. Employees cannot be charged for vaccines.

99   Staff can put themselves at risk of blood-borne infection if they resheath needles following contact with a service user. Needles should not be resheathed after use but disposed of directly into a sharps container (see 'Clinical waste' earlier in this section).

Moving and handling

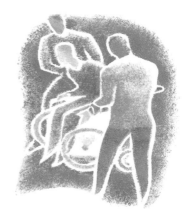

100 The Manual Handling Operations Regulations 1992[17] were introduced to reduce the numbers of injuries from moving and handling throughout industry including the care sector. The term manual handling includes lifting, moving, putting down, pushing, pulling and carrying by hand or bodily force of goods, equipment and people.

The Manual Handling Regulations - key duties

The employer must:
- avoid moving and handling where there is a risk of staff being injured, as far as reasonably practicable;
- assess the risk of injury from moving and handling that cannot be avoided;
- reduce the risk of injury from moving and handling, as far as reasonably practicable.

Employees must:
- make full and proper use of the systems of work provided.

101 If you are looking to avoid moving and handling, consider whether:
- the job is necessary;
- it can be done in a different way (breaking heavy loads into smaller units, enabling the service user to be independent);
- it can be mechanised.

102 In assessing the risk of injury, assess the task and identify ways of reducing the risk by:
- adding specialist sliders or wheels to furniture that has to be moved;
- use of hoists, sliding sheets, turning circles and other devices for moving and handling people;
- providing sack trucks or trolleys;
- spread moving and handling tasks throughout the day.

103 Adopt the measures identified in the assessments to reduce the risk of injury to the lowest reasonably practicable level.

Making an assessment

104 It should be possible to complete the majority of assessments in-house as you know your business better than anyone. Simple tasks only require simple assessments, eg dividing large boxes of stores into smaller loads. More complex tasks will require detailed assessment and will need to be recorded. To save effort you can group common tasks together and then carry out a generic assessment. The assessments should consider the task, the load, the working environment and the individual's capabilities.

The task

105 You need to ask yourself whether the task involves:
- holding the load at a distance from the trunk of the body;
- bending, twisting, stooping or stretching;
- moving the load over excessive distances;
- frequent or prolonged physical effort;
- risk of sudden movement of the load; or
- insufficient rest or recovery periods.

106 Fatigue increases the likelihood of moving and handling injuries and therefore the number and length of rests or recovery periods are important. Work should be organised so that, where practical, moving and handling tasks are spread among staff and throughout the shift. This allows staff longer recovery periods between moving and handling activities. Staffing levels will also affect workloads, rest and recovery periods.

107 Team handling can help some moving and handling problems but it relies on co-ordination of effort, good communication and control. It can create problems so ideally mechanical aids should be used.

108 All equipment should be well maintained. In addition, the Lifting Operations and Lifting Equipment Regulations 1998[18] require that lifting equipment for people (hoists and lifts) are thoroughly examined every six months, unless a scheme of thorough examination is devised by a competent person. This is usually an insurance engineer.

The load

109   The shape and size of inanimate loads affect how difficult they are to lift; so does the stability of the contents, whether they are sharp or hot or there are any grips or handles. The risk of injury may be reduced by redesigning loads/tasks to make them more manageable, ie making them lighter, smaller, easier to grasp, more stable and less damaging to hold.

110   You need to ask yourself whether the load is:
- a person or inanimate object;
- heavy or bulky (if a person whether there is anything they can do to help);
- difficult to grasp;
- physically unstable or involving unpredictable behaviour;
- harmful, eg sharp or hot.

111   Some service users may become violent or agitated when being moved. Others, although willing to assist at the start of manoeuvre, may suddenly find themselves unable to continue. The response by the staff may determine whether injury to themselves or the service users is avoided. Training for staff on how to deal with such situations may help to prevent injury. A natural reaction, while assisting a service user to walk, for example, is to try to prevent them from falling, and injuries have occurred to both staff and service users in such circumstances. If they are properly positioned, the helper may either prevent a fall or allow a controlled slide. Then, having made the service user comfortable, they can determine how to move the service user safely preferably with a mechanical aid.

112   Special techniques may be required for moving and handling service users depending on the situation and the ability of the individual. Care should be taken to avoid tender and painful areas. It is important to remember their dignity, tell them about the equipment and explain how it will be used. Relatives may also need explanation and reassurance about moving and handling equipment.

113   You may need specialist advice on how to help service users in and out of baths, from bed to chair and how to help a service user from the floor after a fall etc. Groups such as the Chartered Society for Physiotherapists, Ergonomic Society, and Royal Society for the Prevention of Accidents (ROSPA) may give further advice on aspects of moving and handling.

114   Service users may suffer from inappropriate handling. Their needs and abilities can change over the course of a day so it may be necessary to reassess service users frequently. It is good practice to include the moving and handling assessments in individual care plans or profiles. The assessment should be available to all workers caring for the service user.

115   The most useful assessments are set out in a simple format so that it is possible to quickly assimilate what equipment, techniques and numbers of staff are appropriate for a service user's needs. A good plan will cover both daytime and night-time care, focusing in on key moves including:
- individual details, including identification, height and weight;
- the extent of the individual's ability to support his or her own weight and any other relevant factors, for example pain, disability, spasm, fatigue, or tendency to fall;
- problems with comprehension, co-operational behaviour;
- recommended methods of movement for the relevant tasks such as sitting, going to the toilet, bathing, transfers and movement in bed;
- details of equipment needed;
- the minimum number of staff required to help;
- other relevant risk factors.

The working environment

116   You need to ask yourself whether there are:
- basic constraints preventing good posture, eg lack of space especially by baths, beds or chairs, height of furniture;
- inadequate or insufficient storage facilities;
- uneven, slippery or unstable floors, carpets impeding free movement of hoists etc;
- changes in floor levels, eg slopes, stairs.

117   Moving and handling tasks are often made easier by good design. For example, employees are often required to care for service users in bed and providing adjustable height beds can help prevent the risks of back injuries. Raising the height of laundry equipment, eg washing machines or driers, by placing

it on a platform can also reduce bending and stooping. Other measures to reduce the amount of handling by care staff are:

- raising the height of beds and chairs using wooden blocks;
- handrails at strategic heights adjacent to the bath and toilet;
- bath hoists/overhead hoists etc;
- walk-in showers with seats;
- cutting slots in bath panels to allow for mobile hoist wheels to fit underneath a bath fixed against a wall.

Individual factors

118   The moving and handling tasks should be designed, where possible, to suit individuals rather than the individual to fit the task. Effective training has an important part to play in reducing the risks but it is not a substitute for improving the task, the load (where possible) and the working environment.

119   Particular consideration should be given to employees who are pregnant (or have been recently) or those who are known to have injuries or ill health. This may include reassessing the task, the organisation of work, job sharing, relocation, suspension on full pay etc.

120   Training should be appropriate for the job. For instance, a care assistant will require training in all aspects of moving and handling inanimate loads and people. Catering, domestic and maintenance staff will need to concentrate moving and handling inanimate objects. Provision should be made for refresher training of staff and the frequency of this should be assessed according to the risks. Staff moving and handling people may need to have annual refresher training, whereas in other situations it may be acceptable to have refresher training every few years.

121   Clothing, uniforms, footwear and protective equipment are other factors that have direct impact on movement and the ability to choose the appropriate posture while moving and handling. They should allow staff to perform a full range of movement.

122   The HSE guide on the Manual Handling Operations Regulations 1992[17] contains more details of factors to consider during an assessment.

Recording moving and handling assessments

123   The assessment should be recorded unless:
- it could be very easily repeated and explained at any time because it is simple and obvious;
- the manual handling operation is quite straightforward, low-risk, going to last a short time and time taken to record it would be disproportionate to the risk.

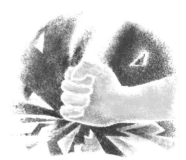

Aggression and violence to staff

124   Employers are beginning to recognise that aggression/violence to staff at work can be a source of injury and distress. The term violence covers a wide range of incidents, not all of which involve injury. The definition adopted in this publication is: 'any incident in which a person working in a care home is verbally abused, threatened or assaulted by a service user or a member of the public in circumstances relating to his or her employment'.

Examples

A carer is bitten by a person with learning disabilities in the course of the normal care of that person.

A manager is verbally abused by an irate visitor who considers that his relative has not been properly treated.

A carer is verbally abused and threatened by a service user who is unwilling to take prescribed medication.

A contractor repairing an item of equipment is punched by a confused service user.

125   Managing violence to staff is covered by the general duties of the HSW Act and the Management of Health and Safety at Work Regulations 1999. Employers and staff should not accept aggression/violence as an unavoidable occupational hazard but establish systems to prevent or reduce aggressive behaviour to employees by service users, their relatives or friends. The best way to tackle violence is for employers and employees to work together.

126   You need to establish if there is a problem with aggression/violence in your home by undertaking a risk assessment using the five steps format (see 'Risk assessment' section). Part of the assessment could include information from incidents and staff perception. You might need to consider particular activities that can trigger aggressive responses, for example a service user who is not permitted to smoke unsupervised and has to wait for a cigarette.

127   If aggressive and violent incidents that do not cause injury are included in the accident and ill health recording system, then this data can be used to identify potential problems. Staff may need encouragement to report these types of incidents as well as those that cause injury.

Precautions

128   There are a number of precautions that can be used in care homes to prevent and control aggression/violence to staff. Not all these measures will be suitable and some will be easier to implement than others. They include changing the following aspects:

Work activities

- Jobs people do and how they are done
- Instructions, verbal or written, for the job
- The system for sharing information about service users/relatives
- Adequate staffing levels according to the risk (including cover for meal breaks, handover periods etc)
- The response to incidents and how they are recorded

Workplace

- Arranging seats in clusters rather than ranks
- Diffused and glare-free lighting
- Subdued wall coverings and surface finishes
- Plants and pictures (firmly fixed to prevent use as weapons)
- Locking buildings when staff are working on their own or at night
- Security systems such as personal units linked to building alarm systems

Communication

- Information passed on at referral
- Provision of information to staff, volunteers, relatives, service users
- Appropriate training to help staff work safely when dealing with potentially aggressive or violent people
- Leaving lists of visits and regular telephone contact for mobile staff

129 If risks from aggression and violence are to be managed successfully, there must be support from those at the top of the organisation. This can be expressed in a clear statement of policy, supported by organisation and arrangements to ensure that statement is implemented. See Figure 1 in the 'Managing health and safety' section.

Developing a policy

130 Policies on violence and aggression need to fit within the framework of the overall health and safety policy. The key elements include:

- recognition of the risks;
- commitment to introducing precautions to reduce that risk;
- a statement of who is responsible for doing what;
- an explanation of what is expected from individual employees;
- a commitment to supporting people who have been assaulted or suffered verbal abuse.

Information and training

131 A flow of information about potentially violent situations within the organisation will help staff assess the likelihood of aggression or violent assault. This is particularly appropriate when:

- new members of staff are involved;
- new service users are admitted;
- there has been a change in a service user's mental or physical state, medication, behaviour, mood etc;
- known violent service users are being transferred to the home.

132 In addition, training in the prevention and management of violence/aggression can provide staff with techniques to reduce or diffuse aggression/violence. It should be available to all employees who come into contact with service users. The training should cover:

- causes of violence;
- recognition of warning signs;
- relevant interpersonal skills;
- details of working practices and control measures;
- incident-reporting procedures.

133 Confidence and capability are important when dealing with a potentially aggressive or violent incident and staff may need refresher training from time to time to update their skills.

134 Establishing a relationship of trust and understanding with the service users will help to ensure that tensions and anxieties are expressed before they reach a stage where they are released through violent behaviour.

Helping staff after an incident

135 It can be useful to bring staff together after an incident to discuss what happened. This process of debriefing may have two functions: to establish details of the event and to provide emotional help. It is sometimes appropriate to supplement debriefing by confidential counselling. Staff morale and confidence may be improved to see that there is a genuine commitment from employers to pursue prosecution in cases of serious assault.

136 More detailed information on managing violence and aggression can be found in *Violence and aggression to staff in health services: Guidance on assessment and management.*[19]

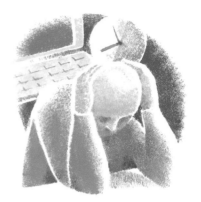

Work-related stress

What is stress?

137   Stress is people's natural reaction to excessive pressure - it isn't a disease. But if stress is excessive and goes on for some time, it can lead to mental and physical ill health, eg depression, nervous breakdown, heart disease. Being under pressure often improves performance and can be a good thing for some people. But when demands and pressures become excessive, they may lead to stress.

138   As an employer, is it your duty to make sure that your employees aren't made ill by their work. Employees can be made ill by stress. The cost of stress to your company may show up as high staff turnover, an increase in sickness absence, reduced work performance, poor timekeeping and more customer complaints. Therefore action to reduce stress can be very cost-effective. Employers who don't take stress seriously may leave themselves open to compensation claims from employees who have suffered ill health from work-related stress. Fortunately, reducing stress need not cost you a lot of money.

Risk assessment

139   Firstly, you need to identify if stress at work is a problem. A risk assessment should identify activities or jobs that give rise to high and long-lasting levels of stress. They should also identify who might be harmed and what you are currently doing to reduce stress levels. It should identify if there are any more actions that could be implemented to decrease stress levels further.

140   You are not under a legal duty to prevent ill health caused by stress due to problems outside work, eg financial or domestic. But non-work problems can make it difficult for people to cope with the pressures of work, and their performance at work might suffer. So being understanding to staff in this position may be in your interest.

141   Many of the outward signs of stress in individuals should be noticeable to managers and colleagues. Look in particular for changes in the person's behaviour, such as deteriorating relationships with colleagues, irritability, indecisiveness, absenteeism or reduced performance. Those suffering from stress may also smoke or drink alcohol more than usual. They might also complain about their health.

142   There is no single best way of handling work-related stress. What you will do will depend on your working practices and causes of the problem. But only providing training or help (or both) for sufferers will not be enough - it will not actually tackle the source of the problem. The following points are some suggestions of how to tackle stress.

Doing the job

Problems that can lead to stress

Working with high-risk service users

Lack of information on service users

Working alone

Inadequate resources and equipment

What management can do

Change the way the jobs are done and move people between tasks

Give staff as much information as possible

Try to give warning of urgent or important jobs, prioritise tasks, stop unnecessary work

Provide relevant training

Responsibilities

Problems that can lead to stress

Poor management

Confusion about roles

Having responsibility for looking after others as part of the job

What management can do

Make sure that everyone has clearly defined objectives and responsibilities

Provide training and support for those with responsibility for management or caring for others

Balancing work and home

Problems that lead to stress
Irregular patterns of workdays

Short notification of workdays

What management can do
See if there is scope for flexible work schedules
(eg flexible working hours)

Plan work rosta well in advance

Relationships

Problems that can lead to stress
Poor relationship with others

Bullying, racial or sexual harassment

What management can do
Provide training in interpersonal skills

Set up effective systems to prevent bullying and
harassment (ensure there is an agreed grievance
procedure and proper investigation of complaints)

Working conditions

Problems that can lead to stress
Physical danger (eg hazardous chemicals, risk of
violence) and poor physical working conditions

What management can do
Provide adequate control measures

Management attitudes

Problems that can lead to stress
Lack of control over work activities

Lack of communication and consultation

Negative culture, eg a culture for blame when things
go wrong, denial of potential problems

Inability to discuss problems because fear of
criticism/reprisals

Lack of support for individuals to develop their skills

What management can do
Provide opportunities for staff to contribute ideas,
especially in planning and organising their own jobs

Introduce clear business objectives, good
communication and close employee involvement,
particularly during periods of change

Be honest with yourself, set a good example, respect
others and listen to them

Provide as much support as possible (eg leave,
financial help) for individuals to develop their skills

143   It is important to involve and consult with staff
at all stages of managing stress. Further information
can be found in *Tackling work-related stress: A
manager's guide to improving and maintaining
employee health and well-being*[20] and in a leaflet
Tackling work-related stress: A guide for employees.[21]

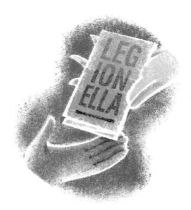

Legionella

144   Legionnaires' disease is a potentially fatal type of pneumonia. It is contracted by inhaling tiny airborne droplets or particles containing viable legionella bacteria. Although healthy individuals may develop legionnaires' disease, there are some people who are more at risk such as the elderly, smokers, alcoholics and those with cancer, diabetes or chronic respiratory or kidney disease.

145   Legionella bacteria are common and can be found in water systems, wet air conditioning plant, whirlpool baths and hydrotherapy baths. They favour water temperatures in the range of 20-45°C to multiply. Proliferation is not likely below 20°C and they will not survive above 60°C. Water services should therefore be operated at temperatures that prevent growth:

*   Hot water storage (calorifiers) should be maintained at more than 60°C.
*   Hot water should be distributed at least at 50°C.
*   Cold water should be stored and distributed at 20°C or below.
*   The water system should be routinely checked and inspected by a competent person, in accordance with the risk assessment.

146   Water stagnation can encourage conditions that favour the growth of legionella. It is therefore advisable to remove dead runs in pipework from the system, flush out seldom-used shower heads, taps and remaining deadlegs periodically (weekly), and to remove any dirt and limescale. Water systems can be designed to avoid the conditions that favour growth of legionella. These are:

*   ensuring that the pipe work is as short and direct as possible;
*   ensuring adequate insulation of pipes and tanks;
*   using materials that do not encourage the growth of legionella;
*   protecting against contamination, eg fitting storage tanks with lids.

147   If hot water is not required for laundry etc then you might wish to consider the use other methods for controlling legionella, eg ionisation, ultraviolet light, chlorine dioxide, ozone treatment or regular thermal disinfection. Their application will need suitable assessment as part of the overall water treatment programme including proper installation, maintenance and monitoring (to be able to demonstrate that bacteria counts are below the acceptable level).

148   More detailed information inspection and maintenance of systems can be found in the Approved Code of Practice and guidance on legionnaires' disease.[22]

Water temperatures and hot surfaces

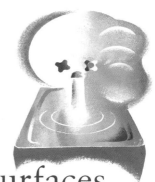

Scalding

149 Homes have increased water temperatures for a number of reasons but mainly to satisfy hot water demand and efficient running of the boiler rather than to control legionella. High water temperatures create a scalding risk. When water temperatures are in excess of 44°C, there is a high risk of burns and scalds to the elderly, people with mental illness or learning disabilities, children, anyone with reduced sensitivity to temperature or anyone who cannot react appropriately, or quickly enough, to prevent injury. Unfortunately, many of these accidents have been fatal.

150 These fatal accidents have mainly occurred when service users have been either taking a bath or a shower. It is essential that where vulnerable people are at risk from scalding during whole body immersion water temperatures do not exceed 44°C. The Department of Health has drawn up guidelines specifying maximum 'safe' hot water temperatures for a range of applications; these are set out in the NHS Estates guidance note on safe hot water and surface temperatures.[23]

Precautions

151 If bathing facilities are accessible by vulnerable service users then the following set of steps should be taken:

- **Fitting of thermostatic mixing valves (type 3)** - to prevent water at greater than 44°C (showers should not exceed 41°C) being discharged from taps where there is potential for whole body immersion. It is particularly important that thermostatic mixing valves (TMVs) are maintained to the standard recommended by the manufacturer as there have been fatal accidents where homes have not maintained valves adequately. A documented maintenance schedule should be followed.

- **Adequate training and supervision** - to ensure that staff involved in bathing service users understand the risks and precautions. This will include filling the bath and checking the temperature before the person gets into it and also periodic (eg weekly) monitoring of the outlet temperature of the bath/shower water using a bath thermometer. If it is necessary to add hot water while the person is in the bath, this should be done slowly and the water should be tested as it is added. If water exceeds 44°C from the tap, staff should report this to the person in charge and access to the bath/shower concerned restricted until such time as repairs or other remedial action have been carried out. Unfortunately, service users have been fatally scalded by being lowered by care staff into baths which were too hot.

- **Risk assessments** - need to take into account the vulnerability of all those who have access to the bathing facilities. The results of these assessments may be recorded in the individual service user care plans, which should include an assessment of the capabilities and should specify whether a service user is able to bathe themselves unsupervised. Questions to be asked may include:
  - Can the service user get in/out, sit up and/or wash themselves unaided?
  - Is the service user's sensitivity to temperature impaired?
  - Is the service user's mental state such that they can recognise the bath is too hot?
  - Is the service user capable of summoning assistance if needed?
  - Will any lifting or other aids limit the service user's mobility in the bath?
  - Is the service user liable to try and run themselves a bath or add water when unattended? (This is a particular issue for confused people and those with dementia.)

152   Other steps - such as locking bathroom doors or the removal of hot tap heads - should only be used as a temporary measure as they rely on staff following a system of work.

153   In rehabilitation training areas the object is to provide a near-domestic environment. Blending and temperature control devices are unlikely to be needed provided that there is an adequate supervision by staff who have received information and training on the risks of scalding and the safe procedures to be adopted. Labelling hot water outlets with 'very hot water' signs will help to prevent inadvertent scalding. Other regulatory bodies may require temperature control devices to be fitted in certain circumstances.

Hot surfaces

154   High temperatures of circulating water in heating and domestic hot water systems have also given rise to serious injuries and fatalities from contact with hot pipes or radiators. Where there is a risk of a vulnerable person sustaining a burn from a hot surface, eg radiator or pipe, then the surface should not exceed 43°C when the system is running at the maximum design output. The options for ensuring safety include:

• providing low surface temperature heat emitters, eg cool wall radiators;
• guarding the heated areas, eg providing radiator covers, covering exposed pipe work;
• reducing the flow temperatures.

155   Other design solutions that ensure the maximum surface temperature does not exceed 43°C are acceptable.

156   Where alterations are necessary, priority should be given to those radiators where service users are most likely to sustain an injury, such as bedrooms and bathrooms.

Accident cases

A 65-year-old man living in a private nursing home died after being lowered into a hot bath by two nurses who had not checked the temperature of the water.

A woman fell against a hot radiator and couldn't get up. She sustained serious burns and died one week later.

A man with learning disabilities climbed into a bath that had been run for him. He suffered serious burns as a result of extremely hot water. The bath had been fitted with a thermostatic mixing valve but it had not been maintained. Temperature recordings of the bath had been made but no one had highlighted the problem of extremely high temperatures.

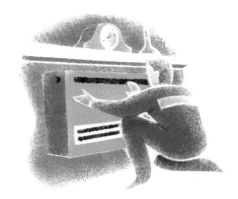

Utilities

Gas

157   The Gas Safety (Installation and Use) Regulations 1998[24] apply to all gas appliances in care homes. Gas appliances, together with the pipe work and flues, should be checked for safety at least once a year. Servicing at the same time is advisable to make sure they are maintained in a safe, efficient condition. Any work on gas appliances and pipe work must be undertaken by companies or individuals who are members of the Council for Registered Gas Installers (CORGI).

Electricity

158   Electricity can kill. It also causes shock and burns, and can start fires. Even non-fatal shocks can cause severe and permanent injury. Those using electrical equipment may not be the only ones at risk. Most accidents can be avoided by careful planning and straightforward precautions.

159   The use of electricity in care homes is primarily covered by the Electricity at Work Regulations 1989.[25] These Regulations require employers and self-employed people to maintain, so far as is reasonably practicable, electrical systems and electrical equipment within their control. Electrical systems include the lighting and power circuits; electrical equipment will include appliances such as washing machines, vacuum cleaners, irons, food preparation machinery etc.

160   In care homes the main electrical hazards are:
- contact with live parts causing shock and burns (normal mains voltage 230 volts AC, and in some circumstances even lower voltages can kill); and
- faults that could cause fires.

161   Work on electrical equipment, eg installation work, inspection, testing and maintenance, must only be done by someone who is competent to do it. This means they should have the appropriate technical knowledge and practical experience to prevent danger. Work can be carried out by care home employees provided they are competent. If you are using an outside contractor, one possible way of indicating competence would be to select an organisation which is a member of a recognised electrical contracting trade body, such as the National Inspection Council for Electrical Installation Contracting (NICEIC) or the Electrical Contractors Association (ECA).

Fixed electrical installation

162   Fixed electrical installation should be designed and installed to a suitable standard. The most widely used standard in the UK is BS 7671: 1992 *Requirements for electrical installations*. This is also known as the Institution of Electrical Engineers (IEE) Wiring Regulations, although they are not statutory regulations. The IEE recommends that fixed electrical installation should be inspected and tested at regular intervals; for care homes this would normally be at least every five years. Inspection and testing should be carried out by a competent person who should advise of any defects, repair them or produce a report indicating what needs to be done to remedy them. Serious defects should be remedied as soon as possible. The possession of a defect report and suitable defects remedy system is one way of indicating compliance (in respect of maintenance for the installation) with the Electricity at Work Regulations.

Portable equipment

163   A simple, inexpensive system of looking for visible signs of damage or faults on electrical equipment should help control electrical risks.

164   The first step of such a system is the user check. Frequent, regular in-house visual checks of equipment should be carried out to ensure cables are in good condition, plugs are correctly connected and the equipment is generally in good repair. These checks can be undertaken by the users before and during use, provided they are competent to do so. Where equipment is protected by a residual current device (RCD), then the RCD will also need to be adequately maintained.

165 Staff should be encouraged to report any evident electrical problem, for example broken plugs, frayed flex, discoloured or overheated cables. Defective or unsuitable equipment should be immediately withdrawn from service until it is either repaired or destroyed.

166 The next step is to set in place a formal system of a more in-depth visual inspection of equipment. Staff who have received the necessary training may be able to check the fuse rating or the earth connections as part of this inspection.

167 Some equipment belonging to service users may also need to be inspected since it can have an impact on the safety of others in the home, especially care staff and housekeepers. There should always be an initial visual check when items are first brought into the premises.

168 Some electrical testing may be necessary to ensure that equipment is safe. Portable equipment (such as vacuum cleaners and irons) which is subject to constant and heavy use may need more than the occasional visual check to ensure that is it safe and therefore testing would be appropriate. It is clearly sensible to keep records of all inspections and tests carried out on each piece of equipment. Table 8 gives a guide on the frequency of inspection and tests of various items of equipment.

169 Damaged cables should generally be replaced completely. Never carry out makeshift repairs to cables. When joining flexible cables, proper connectors should be used, ie not strip connector blocks.

Outdoor electrical safety

170 All plugs, sockets and connectors used outside should be suitable for outdoor use. Domestic 13 amp plugs and sockets manufactured to BS 1363 are not suitable for use outside. The equipment should be made to BS EN 60309 when marked with IP43 or IP44.

171 The cables of electrical equipment should be inspected before use and kept out of the way of possible hazards caused by the passage of vehicles or the moving blades of grass-cutters.

172 The electricity supply to any hand-held or hand-manipulated electrical equipment used outdoors should be protected by a residual current device (RCD) with a rated tripping current of 30 mA or less and no adjustable time delay. RCDs will not provide protection when a person holds live and neutral cords of a severed cable connected to the supply.

173 Where possible, the RCD should be located at the supply distribution board or at the sockets supplying the equipment. RCD protective plugs or plug-in adapters will provide protection if nothing better is available. Fixed RCDs should comply with BS 4293: 1983, or BS EN 61008-1: 1995.

174 Portable RCDs should comply with BS 7071: 1992. There are some portable electronic RCDs that do not comply with this because they do not have an external test button as they have in-built self-checking features. This type of RCD may still be safe to use. If you are in any doubt, check with a competent person.

175 RCDs can develop faults which are not visible. They are fitted with a test button that should be operated on a regular basis to check the effect of the operation of the device. If the RCD fails to trip when the test button is pressed, it should be taken out of service and replaced. They should be included in the electrical maintenance and inspection system.

176 If an RCD trips frequently for no apparent reason there may be a fault with the RCD or the equipment it is supplying; have both checked by a competent person. Never by-pass on the RCD because it is tripping out, this may be caused by a dangerous fault.

177 For further information on electrical safety, see *Electrical safety and you*.[26] See the 'Outdoor health and safety' section for more information on outdoor hazards.

Table 8 Suggested intervals for checking portable electrical equipment

Equipment/environment	User checks	Formal visual inspection	Combined inspection and testing
Battery operated (less than 20 volts)	No	No	No
Extra low voltage (less than 50 volts AC): Telephone equipment, low voltage desk lights	No	No	No
Information technology: Desk-top computers, VDU screens	No	Yes 2-4 years	No if double insulated - otherwise up to 5 years
Photocopiers, fax machines: Not hand-held. Rarely moved	No	Yes 2-4 years	No if double insulated - otherwise up to 5 years
Double insulated equipment: Not hand-held. Moved occasionally, eg fans, table lamps, slide projectors	No	Yes 2-4 years	No
Double insulated equipment: Hand-held, eg some floor cleaners	Yes	Yes, 6 months-1 year	No
Earthed equipment (Class 1): Electric kettles, some floor cleaners, some kitchen equipment and irons	Yes	Yes, 6 months-1 year	Yes 1-2 years
Cables (leads and plugs connected to the above)

Extension leads (mains voltage) | Yes | Yes, 6 months-4 years depending on the type of equipment it is connected to | Yes, 1-5 years depending on the type of equipment it is connected to |

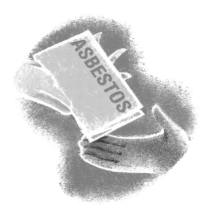

Asbestos

178   If you own, manage or have responsibilities for a workplace building that may contain asbestos, you need to think about the risks of exposure to workers and others who may use the building. It is your job to manage that risk. A sound management strategy will help to ensure that you do not put others at risk.

179   Breathing in air containing asbestos dust can lead to asbestos-related diseases, which are mainly cancer of the chest and lungs. There are no cures for these diseases and the incident rate is rising. People most at risk are associated with the building trade such as caretakers, electricians, plumbers, maintenance workers and carpenters carrying out refurbishment, repairs or maintenance work on buildings which contain asbestos. Other workers, not normally associated with the building trade, may also disturb asbestos. For instance, computer installers (particularly cabling installers), fire alarm installers, window-blind fitters, or telecommunications engineers could be at risk.

180   Asbestos is likely to be present if the building was constructed or refurbished between 1950 and 1980, particularly if it also has a steel frame and/or boilers with thermal insulation.

181   Asbestos can be found in:
- sprayed asbestos and asbestos loose packing - generally used as fire-breaks in ceiling voids;
- moulded or preformed sprayed coatings and lagging - generally used in thermal insulation of pipes and boilers;
- insulating boards used for fire protection, thermal insulation, partitioning and ducts;
- some ceiling tiles;
- asbestos cement products that can be compressed into flat or corrugated sheets (these sheets are largely used as roofing and wall cladding). Other asbestos cement products include gutters, rain water pipes and water tanks;
- certain textured ceilings.

182   Care home owners, managers and maintenance staff need to know the following information about asbestos and this information should be recorded and easily accessible:
- the location of asbestos;
- the form of asbestos (lagging, ceiling tiles, partition board etc);
- the condition of the asbestos; and
- preferably, the type of asbestos (blue, brown or white).

183   You might need to arrange to analyse samples of materials that you suspect contain asbestos. Do not break or damage material that may contain asbestos in an attempt to identify it. Samples should only be taken by suitably trained people, eg from companies accredited by the UK Accreditation Service (UKAS).

Deciding what to do

184   If the asbestos is in good condition, not likely to be damaged and not likely to be worked on, it is safe to leave it in place and introduce the management system. This system should periodically check that the asbestos is correctly labelled, it remains in a good condition and it has not been damaged.

185   If asbestos is in poor condition or it is likely to be damaged or disturbed, it should be repaired, sealed, enclosed or removed. You will need to seek specialist advice from a contractor licensed by HSE on the appropriate action to take.

186   Further advice on dealing with asbestos is available in various HSE publications – see 'Further reading' for details.

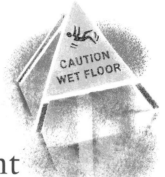

General working environment

187 The Workplace (Health, Safety and Welfare) Regulations 1992[27] are intended to ensure a healthy and safe working environment, and to ensure that adequate welfare facilities are provided for people at work.

The Workplace Regulations - main topics

- Initial structure of the building as it affects users, eg design of windows to allow safe cleaning, stairs.
- The interaction between the building, its layout and the people using it as a workplace, eg provisions for ventilation, traffic routes.
- The provision of basic facilities for employees, eg toilets and rest rooms.

Floors

188 The majority of workplace injuries are as a result of slips, trips and falls so particular attention should be paid to ways of preventing them. It is important that floor coverings are appropriate to the environment but, where possible, slip-resistant surfaces are advisable. In addition, flat floor surfaces that are free from obstructions will help to reduce the likelihood of such accidents.

189 A system to minimise the amount of wet floor area and warning signs should be used when washing hard floor surfaces.

190 Holes and defects in floor coverings should be repaired promptly, particularly those on staircases. Where immediate repair cannot be made, it may be necessary to prevent people passing through the area by cordoning it off.

191 The use of strategically placed handrails offers the service user security, especially where there are changes of floor levels.

Stairs

192 Stairs can present a hazard to everyone. They should be in a safe condition, kept free of obstructions and well lit.

193 It is advisable that stairs should not be steep, winding, curved or have open risers. If service users lack mobility and require extra support, then the stairs should be of adequate width and have handrails on both sides of the stairway.

194 It may be appropriate for some stairs to have restricted access, eg locking the door to steep cellar stairs. Before fitting locks to other doors it is advisable to talk to your registration and inspection unit and the fire prevention officer.

Accident case
An 87-year-old service user sustained fatal injuries when he fell down a staircase. He opened a door leading immediately to a cellar stairway.

Windows

195 Serious injuries have occurred when people have fallen through glass windows. It may therefore be necessary to fit suitable safety film (or replace with safety glazing to BS 6262) to glass at or below waist level. As an alternative, a barrier may be provided to raise the effective height of the sill.

196 Glass doors and patio windows must be fitted with toughened or safety glass or covered with a protective film that prevents glass from shattering. They must have a conspicuous mark or feature sufficiently obvious that people will be unlikely to collide with them. When replacement glass is required then reference to BS 6262 should be made.

197 Any windows that are accessible to vulnerable service users (2 m above ground level), can be opened and are large enough to allow people to fall out should be restrained sufficiently to prevent such falls. It is advisable to restrict the opening to 100 mm (based on NHS guidance). Double-hung, sash-type windows can be easily and cheaply modified to reduce the size

Health and safety in care homes

of the opening by screwing wood blocks into the sash boxes. Casement windows can be restricted by fitting a chain between the frame and the opening light. Any restraining device and fixings should be strong enough to withstand damage.

198   Any window alterations should be discussed with the Fire Prevention Officer.

> **Accident cases**
>
> A 91-year-old service user fell 3 m from her bedroom window and died from her injuries. The window could be fully opened.
>
> A 63-year-old service user fell to her death from her first-floor window. The window was of a hung-sash type.

Doors

199   Doors should be designed so they can be opened easily by staff and service users. Where service users are frail, doors fitted with strong self-closers should be avoided. In some instances, where it does not cause an obstruction, it might be beneficial to re-hang some doors to open outwards, eg in toilets and bathrooms, as this improves access for emergencies and for moving and handling.

200   Where doors (and gates) swing in both directions, a transparent panel should be provided.

Lifts

201   All new passenger lifts should be constructed to a suitable standard (for example BS EN 81 *Safety rules for the construction and installation of lifts* - Part 1: *Electric lifts* or Part 2: *Hydraulic lifts*), and must comply with The Lifts Regulations 1997 and Lifting Operations and Lifting Equipment Regulations 1998.

202   Passenger lifts installed in existing homes that have been built in accordance with BS 5900, known as 'home lifts', should be upgraded where possible. Many of these lifts will be nearing the end of their operational life. They should be replaced by lifts complying with the BS EN 81 series or a design that gives an equivalent level of protection.

203   The Lifting Operations and Lifting Equipment Regulations 1998[18] require that personal lifting

equipment (hoists and lifts for people) are thoroughly examined every six months unless a separate thorough examination scheme is devised by a competent person. It may be necessary to inspect the equipment in-between thorough examinations. The competent person would usually be an insurance company surveyor or engineer from the lift company who specialises in this work. The competent person should provide the proprietor with a report of the results of the examination of the lift. It is advisable that these records are kept available for inspection at the home.

204   In addition to undergoing the thorough examination, lifts and hoists must be adequately maintained in accordance with the manufacturer's instructions. The manufacturer's instructions should also be followed regarding the safe and proper operation of the lift; this is particularly important with hydraulic lifts.

205   Some automatic lift doors close quickly and/or the closing mechanism is too strong for some service users, especially those who are unable to enter or leave the lift cage quickly, resulting in the service user being knocked or trapped by the door. Altering the door closing mechanism so that it closes slowly and less forcefully may help to prevent accidents. Maximum limits for energy and speed of doors are given in Clause 8.7 of BS EN 81-1 and 2.

206   You should follow the manufacturer's advice on the safe release of passengers from a lift car in an 'emergency' situation. In the event of trained staff not being available, then the lift maintenance company should be contacted. On no account should untrained staff attempt to free passengers trapped in a lift car.

Stair lifts

207   Stair lifts should be manufactured to ISO 9386 *Power-operated platforms for persons with impaired mobility - Rules for safety, dimensions and functional operation*. Part 2: *Powered stair lifts for seated, standing and wheelchair users moving in an inclined plane*, or the equivalent European harmonised standard.

208   Stair lifts should not normally be installed in new care homes since they are designed for use in domestic premises where only infrequent or light use of the stair lift normally occurs. However, in some circumstances they may be used in commercial premises provided that the additional features specified in Annex G of ISO 9386 and BS 5776: 1996 Appendix A are followed, namely:

- stair lifts should be installed in care homes only in exceptional circumstances and only where it is not reasonably practicable to incorporate a passenger lift;
- in no circumstances should a stair lift be considered to be a suitable means of escape;
- before installing a stair lift, there should be full consultation with:
  - the Fire Prevention Officer to ensure the proposal will not conflict with means of escape provisions and evacuation procedures;
  - your enforcing authority office to ensure compliance with relevant health and safety requirements;
  - the building control department of the local authority to ensure compliance with the relevant building regulations;
  - the registration and inspection unit to ensure compliance with relevant registration requirements;
- appropriate safety signs and instructions for use should be clearly displayed at each end of travel.

209   If the staff operate the stair lift, a competent person should thoroughly examine it every six months or in accordance with an examination scheme. The stair lift should be adequately maintained in accordance with the manufacturer's instructions and inspected at appropriate intervals between thorough examinations.

210   Service users should be assessed to ascertain whether they are able to use the stair lift safely without assistance. Where service users require help in using the stair lift, staff should be trained in its use and the best way to assist the service user.

Vertical lifting platforms

211   Vertical lifting platforms for use by disabled persons should be manufactured to ISO 9386 Part 1: *Vertical lifting platforms*. They are not designed to replace conventional lifts but to by-pass short flights of stairs where it would not be practical to install a conventional lift. The scope of the ISO 9386-1 limits the maximum vertical travel to 4 m and the speed to 0.15 m per second.

212   Advice on the design, construction, installation, operation and maintenance of vertical lifting platforms is provided in BS 6440: 1999 *Powered lifting platforms for use by disabled persons - Code of practice.*

Accommodation for clothing

213   Accommodation should be provided for any employees' own clothing that is not worn during working hours, and for special clothing that is worn by any person at work but which is not taken home, eg overalls provided by the employer.

214   Where clothing has to be changed at work, changing facilities should be provided. These should either be separate facilities for men and women or for individual use/different times.

Staff rest rooms

215   Care homes must have a separate rest room for the use of employees. Rest rooms must be large enough, and have sufficient chairs and tables for the number of employees likely to use them at any one time. Where meals are regularly eaten in the workplace, there should be a place for staff to eat. Suitable arrangements are also necessary to protect non-smokers from discomfort caused by tobacco smoke.

216   Suitable facilities must be provided for pregnant workers or nursing mothers to rest. This could be a couch in a first-aid room or a bed in an unoccupied room.

Smoking

217   There is increasing concern over the possible health effects of breathing other people's tobacco smoke - environmental tobacco smoke (ETS). Work is

one of a few situations where non-smokers may have to spend long periods in close contact with smokers.

218   Employers should consider drawing up a policy to limit ETS at work. There is the added complication of the care home not only being a workplace but also a home where service users should have certain freedoms as if in their own private dwelling. Full consultation with employees and service users is highly desirable for the smooth implementation of policies designed to limit exposure to ETS. A policy is very much more likely to be accepted by employees and service users if they feel they have been properly consulted.

219   An effective policy on smoking may include the following elements:

- allocating smokers and non-smokers separate rooms where possible;
- designating separate smoking and non-smoking common rooms;
- banning smoking in all common areas such as corridors, lifts and dining rooms;
- improving ventilation/extraction systems so that smoke is more effectively removed from the working environment.

220   Some service users may wish to smoke in their bedrooms. Individual risk assessments should be completed before seeking the views of the Fire Prevention Officer.

Toilets and washing facilities

221   Suitable and sufficient toilets and washing facilities be provided for the maximum number of people likely to be at work at any one time (see table below). Means for disposal of sanitary dressings should be provided where toilets are used by women.

Number of persons at work	Numbers of toilets	Number of wash basins
1-5	1	1
6-25	2	2
26-50	3	3

222   Generally, staff should have separate toilet facilities to those provided for residents. However, in small homes where space is at a premium this may not be practicable. Where facilities are shared, the number of toilets and washing facilities should be increased if necessary. Environmental Health Departments may insist on separate toilet facilities for kitchen staff for food hygiene reasons.

Kitchen health and safety

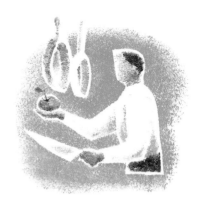

223 Kitchens in care homes vary from domestic-type kitchens in small homes, where service users take some part in preparing their own meals, to commercially designed kitchens that are fully equipped to meet the needs of a large home.

224 You should contact the environmental health department of your local authority for information on food hygiene.

Layout

225 The layout of the kitchen will depend upon its area and the items of equipment in it. There should always be enough room around equipment for staff and service users to move safely without bumping into each other.

226 There should be enough room to move trolleys, carry trays and hot food. This is particularly important around equipment that has an exposed hot surface, for example a griddle top. Attention to manual handling techniques is particularly important in kitchens where loads and surfaces may be hot and floors wet.

227 People using knives and other hand tools should have enough space to work safely. There have been incidents when one person has accidentally stabbed another because they were working in cramped conditions.

228 Side-hinged and bottom-hinged doors that open just above floor-level should not obstruct a gangway.

229 Hazards can be created by placing some items of equipment next to others, for example a deep-fat-fryer next to a sink, or a shelf above an open-top cooking range.

230 In most care homes, suitably placed windows that are capable of being easily opened and closed may be sufficient for effective ventilation. For kitchens and laundries, that can be hot and humid, consideration should be given to installing mechanical exhaust ventilation.

Floors

231 Slips are the main cause of accidents in kitchens. A slip-resistant floor surface should be provided in kitchens and serveries. The floor should be in a good condition and kept clean. Spillages should be cleaned up immediately and warning signs displayed (see 'General working environment' section).

Equipment

232 All catering equipment should be installed on a level surface and on a secure base. Mobile equipment with fitted castors should have the brakes regularly checked to make sure they are working properly. Smaller pieces of equipment that sit on a worktop should be stable and positioned so that they cannot be dislodged.

233 Some types of equipment, such as food-slicers, mincers, food-processors etc, have dangerous parts and should be fitted with guards to protect the user. Guards should be checked before the equipment is used and maintained in good order. A visual examination should be made and any broken or missing guards should be repaired or replaced. Anyone using such equipment should receive appropriate training.

234 Catering equipment has to be stripped down for cleaning. The equipment should be isolated from the electrical supply before cleaning commences. It should be possible to clean guards easily and thoroughly and they should be replaced after cleaning. Equipment should not be run if any guard has been removed.

Use of pesticides in kitchens

235 If pesticides need to be used then they must be approved for use in the kitchen area. They should only be used according to the instructions on the label and packaging, and COSHH will apply (see section on 'Outdoor health and safety'). Care should be taken to prevent contamination but, where it is suspected, the item should be cleaned before being used again.

When pesticides are applied by pest control operators, employers should liaise with them for advice on the product(s) used, when the treated area can be re-entered, and the precautions to be taken etc.

Laundry health and safety

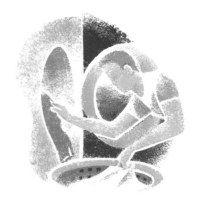

Machinery

236   In most care homes the washing machines and tumble dryers are used extensively, and in some homes by service users as well as staff. The machine suppliers or manufacturers should give you information on maintenance, cleaning of equipment, electrical safety, prevention of fire hazards and turning off water and electrical supplies to the machines in the event of an emergency. Maintenance should be carried out by a competent person.

237   The movement of machinery parts can pose a hazard to staff and service users, so machines should be fitted with an interlock mechanism that prevents them from being set in motion until the front-loading door is closed and this should keep it closed until any accessible moving parts have come to rest. Top-loading machines can be opened during agitation but the machine should be fitted with devices that prevent the transition from agitation to spin until the lid is closed and that keep it closed until the moving parts have stopped.

238   With tumble and spin dryers it is equally important to ensure that opening the door cuts off the electrical supply, bringing the cylinder to a halt. The electrical interlock switch used for this purpose should also prevent powered rotation of the drum until the door is closed.

239   A member of staff should be designated to carry out periodic checks on the interlocking devices on the machines. This can be done simply by trying to start the machines with the doors open and also attempting to open the doors while they are running. A reporting system should be set up so that any user noticing that the machine continues to run after the door has been opened, or there any other defects, passes this information to the person in charge.

240   There is a high risk of fire if the lint traps are not cleaned frequently on tumble dryers. The best way of cleaning these traps is to use a vacuum cleaner as this minimises the dust exposure to the laundry staff and the quantity of dust released into the atmosphere.

Mechanical exhaust ventilation may be required in laundries that are hot and humid.

241   If bulk detergents etc are used then you need to consider the siting of the containers so that they do not present a moving and handling problem when they require changing. Some concentrated liquid detergents are caustic and therefore covered by COSHH. Staff should be given training in safe handling of the products and protective equipment, eg gloves, goggles or visor.

Handling soiled laundry

242   Procedures should be laid down for the handling of soiled laundry. Soiled laundry should be kept separate from other dirty laundry and should be identified as such, so that suitable precautions (wearing waterproof gloves and an apron) can be taken by the laundry staff. If staff are wearing latex gloves for long periods of time, the potential for latex sensitisation should be considered (see 'Latex sensitisation' section for more details). Any exposed cuts or grazes should be covered with a waterproof dressing. A COSHH assessment similar to that for clinical waste should be carried out for soiled laundry.

243   Heavily soiled laundry should be sluiced in a specially designated sluice sink or washing machine with a sluice wash and never in a bath or sink used for washing clothes by hand. Soiled laundry subjected to a hot wash programme of 65°C for 10 minutes, or 71°C for 3 minutes, will reduce any subsequent contamination risk. Soiled laundry can also be placed in red alginate bags which are then placed in the machine. The bags dissolve during the wash, reducing handling risks.

244   A hand basin, together with a hot and cold water supply, bactericidal soap and disposable paper towels sited in the sluice room, will ensure that any contamination that has taken place is easily and quickly removed without the risk of spreading to other areas.

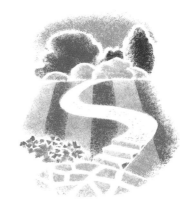

Outdoor health and safety

245   The safety of staff, service users and visitors will extend to garden and outdoor areas. Steps and paths should be kept in good condition and free from obstructions that could lead to tripping hazards, eg refuse and gardening equipment. In winter, gritting and salting steps and paths in anticipation of frost and ice will help to prevent slipping. It may be necessary at times to create a safe pathway through snow. Steps should have a suitable handrail and paths that are used in the hours of darkness should be provided with outdoor lighting (this lighting can be on timer switches or operate on infra red). It may be necessary to establish whether garden ponds, greenhouses, swimming pools and balconies can pose a substantial risk to service users and visitors. A risk assessment should be undertaken which may identify the need to provide some protection against falling in or over these.

Use of powered equipment

246   Protective footwear should be worn when mowing the lawn. It is safer to mow across sloping areas, rather than up and down. When using electric mowers, the cable should be kept out of the way of the mower blade and inspected frequently or prior to use. All plugs, sockets and connectors used in any electric mower cables should be suitable for outdoor use; domestic 13 amp plugs and sockets are not suitable for use in wet or dirty conditions.

247   The electrical supply to any hand-held or hand-manipulated electrical equipment used outdoors should be controlled by a residual current device (RCD). RCDs will offer some protection in the event of a supply cable being severed. The test button on the RCD should be operated on a regular basis to ensure the continued effectiveness of the device. This is because the devices can develop faults that are not visually apparent. For more detail see 'Electricity' in the 'Utilities' section.

248   Petrol mower tanks should be filled outdoors and not in a confined space such as a shed or garage. Petrol should only be kept in containers which are

designed for that purpose. When unclogging or adjusting blades, the machines should always be isolated. This can be achieved by unplugging the electric mower or disconnecting the spark plug on a petrol mower.

Pesticides

249   The term pesticides includes fungicides, herbicides, insecticides, public hygiene pest control products, rodenticides and wood preservatives. Only pesticides that are approved for use in the UK should be used. There is specific legislation that covers the storage and use of pesticides but the Control of Substances Hazardous to Health Regulations 1999 also apply. Guidance is available in the HSE leaflet *Pesticides: Use them safely.*[28] For more detailed information on the legislation and the storage of pesticides contact your enforcing authority.

250   When pesticides are applied by pest control operators, employers should liaise with them for advice on the product(s) used, when the treated area can be used again, and the precautions to be taken, eg preventing access to treated area, closing nearby windows etc.

251   Any person using pesticides should be competent and should have received sufficient instruction, training and guidance to use pesticides safely and legally. The instructions on the label should be rigidly adhered to. Where labels have faded and are unreadable, the pesticide should be disposed of safely. Your supplier (or local waste regulation authorities) can give advice on disposal.

Appendix 1 Self-audit checklist

The following checklist may be used to help direct your attention to areas in the care home which require regular examination. It is by no means an exhaustive list and should be adapted to suit your particular home.

Policies and records

Are they up-to-date, eg health and safety policy, moving and handling policy, lifts, equipment, boiler, accident/incident, staff training?

Is there an accident book?

Do staff know where it is?

Are all reportable accidents reported to the Incident Contact Centre?

Are all assessments (eg general risk assessments, COSHH, manual handling, personal protective equipment) up-to-date?

Are the results implemented in working procedures/practices?

Procedures

Do they need updating?

Is a review of safety policy and management policies required?

Have adequate arrangements for liaising with contractors, employment agencies etc been made?

Are there procedures for consulting with staff and union safety representatives?

Are working time issues resolved?

Staff training

Are all staff trained (including night staff and cleaners)?

Is training adequate and suitable?

Is refresher training provided?

Are all agency staff/contractors informed of policies and procedures?

How is the effectiveness of the training evaluated?

Is sufficient supervision provided?

First aid

Is the first-aid box fully stocked?

Is staff training up-to-date?

COSHH (chemicals)

Are the health hazards from all substances assessed, including those used in the laundry, kitchen, outdoors?

Are control measures implemented?

Are staff trained about safe procedures, use of protective clothing?

Are procedures for spillages in place?

Are new staff trained before using substances?

COSHH (blood-borne diseases)

Have assessments been made, including contaminated/soiled laundry?

Are staff trained in safe working procedures?

Are safe procedures implemented and followed?

Are staff given appropriate protective equipment/clothing and is it used?

Are cuts, grazes etc always covered with waterproof dressings?

Are basic hygiene procedures in place, including regular handwashing?

Are there procedures for cleaning up spillages?

Do staff know what to do in an accident (encourage bleeding, liberally wash wound with soap and water, report and record accident)?

Are staff offered hepatitis B immunisation?

Clinical waste

Is all clinical waste properly bagged in yellow bags\containers?

Is clinical waste segregated from general waste?

Are sharps disposed of in properly constructed sharps containers?

Is the waste storage area safe, secure, clean and tidy?

Is waste regularly collected and disposed of at suitable facilities?

Are there procedures to deal with spillages?

Drugs

Are cupboards locked?

Are service users' drugs in locked cupboard in bedroom?

Moving and handling

Is moving and handling avoided where possible, eg by providing lifting aids or altering work methods?

Have all manual handling tasks been assessed for risks and preventative measures implemented?

Do assessments cover the load, work method, workplace, working environment and individual capability?

Are appropriate lifting aids available and used?

Is equipment, eg beds, adjustable where possible?

Are all staff trained in use of equipment and handling techniques as appropriate?

Are there sufficient staff to carry out work?

Violence

Is there a reporting system in place?

Do staff know how to report incidents and are they encouraged to do so?

Is an assessment of risks of violence made and problems identified?

Have a range of preventative measures been considered (eg environment, staffing, personal security, training)?

Are preventative measures implemented?

Is effectiveness of measures monitored?

Stress

Is there a policy?

Have risk assessments been completed?

Have the preventative/remedial measures been implemented and do they work?

Have staff been involved?

Floors

Are there slippery surfaces?

Have spillages been cleaned up?

Are carpets frayed, flat, even?

Are floor surfaces suitable, non-slip, flat, properly maintained?

Are there obstructions, tripping hazards?

Stairs

Are they well-lit?

Is the stair covering in good condition and clean?

Are there obstructions?

Lighting

Are all bulbs working?

Are lighting levels sufficient?

Are lighting levels sufficient including those on corridors and stairs?

Ventilation

Are there odours?

Are there draughts?

Is there sufficient fresh air?

Have chemicals, fumes, steam/condensation been removed?

Windows

Are restraints in place?

Is glazing in good condition?

Is the glazing material appropriate?

Protective equipment

Is protective equipment (eg gloves, aprons, overalls, goggles) suitable, safe, comfortable?

Is it appropriate, properly stored, cleaned and maintained?

Are staff trained to use it?

Display screen equipment

Has the workstation been analysed and assessed to reduce the risk?

Have the work environment, equipment, furniture, software, individual needs been considered?

Are eye and eyesight tests needed?

Are staff trained to use and set up their VDU workstation safely?

Water and surface temperatures

Are thermostatic mixing valves operating at required temperature?

Are the hot water temperatures regularly tested (using a thermometer)?

Is a maintenance schedule followed for the thermostatic valves?

Are radiators and pipework in excess of 43°C?

If yes, what remedial action has been taken to protect vulnerable service users?

Is the temperature comfortable (not too hot or cold)?

Electrical safety

Have the electrical systems (lighting and power circuits) been checked?

Are appliances in good condition?

Are plugs, sockets, leads in good condition?

Are there trailing leads?

Are appliances correctly fused?

Are there enough sockets (ie sockets not overloaded)?

Are circuit breakers used, eg for lawn mowers?

Are regular checks carried out?

Is equipment taken out of use if faulty and promptly repaired?

Do only competent people check and maintain equipment?

Are staff trained in safe use of equipment?

Welfare

Are there adequate toilet and washing facilities?

Are facilities clean and well maintained?

Is storage provided for staff belongings?

Are staff provided with sufficient rest breaks?

Are smoke-free areas provided?

Is the home regularly cleaned, in good repair and decorative order?

Kitchen safety

Are machines properly guarded?

Are floors clean, slip-resistant and dry?

Is there room to move around safely?

Is ventilation sufficient?

Are staff trained in kitchen hygiene, use of equipment etc?

Is food stored correctly, at correct temperatures etc?

Laundry

Are machine interlocks working?

Is there separation of soiled laundry?

Outside

Are paths and steps in good condition and well lit at night?

Has there been an adequate risk assessment of the risk of falls from balconies and have the findings been implemented?

Are pesticides locked away?

Are staff trained to use outdoor equipment safely?

Do they have suitable protective equipment (identified in the risk assessment)?

Appendix 2 Form F2508 Report of an injury or dangerous occurrence

---

Health and Safety at Work etc Act 1974
The Reporting of Injuries, Diseases and Dangerous Occurrences Regulations 1995

HSE
Health & Safety
Executive

Report of an injury or dangerous occurrence

Filling in this form
This form must be filled in by an employer or other responsible person.

Part A

About you

1 What is your full name?

2 What is your job title?

3 What is your telephone number?

About your organisation

4 What is the name of your organisation?

5 What is its address and postcode?

6 What type of work does the organisation do?

Part B

About the incident

1 On what date did the incident happen?

 /   /

2 At what time did the incident happen?
(Please use the 24-hour clock eg 0600)

3 Did the incident happen at the above address?

Yes ☐ Go to question 4

No ☐ Where did the incident happen?

☐ elsewhere in your organisation – give the name, address and postcode

☐ at someone else's premises – give the name, address and postcode

☐ in a public place – give details of where it happened

If you do not know the postcode, what is the name of the local authority?

4 In which department, or where on the premises, did the incident happen?

F2508 (05.00)

Part C

About the injured person

If you are reporting a dangerous occurrence, go to Part F. If more than one person was injured in the same incident, please attach the details asked for in Part C and Part D for each injured person.

1 What is their full name?

2 What is their home address and postcode?

3 What is their home phone number?

4 How old are they?

5 Are they
☐ male?
☐ female?

6 What is their job title?

7 Was the injured person (tick only one box)
☐ one of your employees?
☐ on a training scheme? Give details:

☐ on work experience?
☐ employed by someone else? Give details of the employer:

☐ self-employed and at work?
☐ a member of the public?

Part D

About the injury

1 What was the injury? (eg fracture, laceration)

2 What part of the body was injured?

Continued overleaf

3 Was the injury (tick the one box that applies)

☐ a fatality?

☐ a major injury or condition? (see accompanying notes)

☐ an injury to an employee or self-employed person which prevented them doing their normal work for more than 3 days?

☐ an injury to a member of the public which meant they had to be taken from the scene of the accident to a hospital for treatment?

4 Did the injured person (tick all the boxes that apply)

☐ become unconscious?

☐ need resuscitation?

☐ remain in hospital for more than 24 hours?

☐ none of the above.

Part E

About the kind of accident

Please tick the one box that best describes what happened, then go to Part G.

☐ Contact with moving machinery or material being machined

☐ Hit by a moving, flying or falling object

☐ Hit by a moving vehicle

☐ Hit something fixed or stationary

☐ Injured while handling, lifting or carrying

☐ Slipped, tripped or fell on the same level

☐ Fell from a height
   How high was the fall?
   [_____] metres

☐ Trapped by something collapsing

☐ Drowned or asphyxiated

☐ Exposed to, or in contact with, a harmful substance

☐ Exposed to fire

☐ Exposed to an explosion

☐ Contact with electricity or an electrical discharge

☐ Injured by an animal

☐ Physically assaulted by a person

☐ Another kind of accident (describe it in Part G)

Part F

Dangerous occurrences

Enter the number of the dangerous occurrence you are reporting. (The numbers are given in the Regulations and in the notes which accompany this form)

[_____]

Part G

Describing what happened

Give as much detail as you can. For instance
• the name of any substance involved
• the name and type of any machine involved
• the events that led to the incident
• the part played by any people.

If it was a personal injury, give details of what the person was doing. Describe any action that has since been taken to prevent a similar incident. Use a separate piece of paper if you need to.

Part H

Your signature

Signature

[_____]

Date

[__ / __ / __]

Where to send the form
Please send it to the Enforcing Authority for the place where it happened. If you do not know the Enforcing Authority, send it to the nearest HSE office.

For official use			
Client number	Location number	Event number	
[_____]	[_____]	[_____]	☐ INV REP ☐ Y ☐ N

Appendix 3 Form F2508A
Report of a case of disease

HSE
Health & Safety
Executive

Health and Safety at Work etc Act 1974
The Reporting of Injuries, Diseases and Dangerous Occurrences Regulations 1995

Report of a case of disease

Filling in this form
This form must be filled in by an employer or other responsible person.

Part A
About you

1 What is your full name?

2 What is your job title?

3 What is your telephone number?

About your organisation

4 What is the name of your organisation?

5 What is its address and postcode?

6 Does the affected person usually work at this address?

Yes ☐ Go to question 7

No ☐ Where do they normally work?

7 What type of work does the organisation do?

Part B
About the affected person

1 What is their full name?

2 What is their date of birth?

/ /

3 What is their job title?

4 Are they
☐ male?
☐ female?

5 Is the affected person (tick one box)
☐ one of your employees?
☐ on a training scheme? Give details:

☐ on work experience?
☐ employed by someone else? Give details:

☐ other? Give details:

F2508A (05.00)

Continued overleaf

Part C

The disease you are reporting

1 Please give:

- the name of the disease, and the type of work it is associated with; or

- the name and number of the disease *(from Schedule 3 of the Regulations – see the accompanying notes).*

2 What is the date of the statement of the doctor who first diagnosed or confirmed the disease?

| / | / |

3 What is the name and address of the doctor?

Continue your description here

Part D

Describing the work that led to the disease

Please describe any work done by the affected person which might have led to them getting the disease.

If the disease is thought to have been caused by exposure to an agent at work *(eg a specific chemical)* please say what that agent is.

Give any other information which is relevant.

Give your description here

Part E

Your signature

Signature

Date

| / | / |

Where to send the form

Please send it to the Enforcing Authority for the place where the affected person works. If you do not know the Enforcing Authority, send it to the nearest HSE office.

For official use

Client number

Location number

Event number

☐ INV   REP   ☐ Y   ☐ N

Health and safety in care homes

49

Appendix 4 Health and safety policy statements

1   Planning for health and safety in a systematic way is the key to achieving acceptable standards, reducing accidents and helping to save operational costs. The company health and safety policy should be a document that helps you realise your plans. It sets out who does what, when and where for health and safety.

Statement of general policy

2   When preparing the health and safety policy, begin by setting out your general aims (the legal responsibility placed upon the company to provide and maintain healthy and safe conditions for all employees and other people who might be affected). Undertake, for example, to:
- provide enough resources for effective implementation of the policy;
- plan systematically;
- revise and develop the policy (it may be helpful to review the policies at regular intervals, eg annually);
- secure the compliance of all employees by the means of instruction, information and training.

3   It will help to demonstrate the company's level of commitment if the statement is signed and dated by the managing director or partner.

Responsibilities

4   Next, set out people's responsibilities for health and safety:
- identify the director with overall responsibility for health and safety;
- specify duties of managers and supervisors stating, for example, which areas of work they cover. It might be adequate in a small care home for the home manager to be responsible for all day-to-day health and safety matters and for consultation with employees;
- give names and roles of key people such as the home's/company's competent person(s);
- allocate responsibility for accident investigation and reporting;

- identify who organises health and safety training and the provision of information;
- identify who liaises with the enforcing authorities;
- identify who to contact, eg a manager if a health and safety problem arises;
- specify employees' responsibilities and actions if they are not fulfilled;
- arrange consultation between management and employees over matters of health and safety (include the membership of any health and safety committee and the frequency of meetings);
- allocate responsibility for maintenance of buildings and plant.

Arrangements for health and safety

5   Your arrangements for health and safety merit considerable thought. They set out how you put into practice the necessary control measures identified by your risk assessment. The arrangements detail how people fulfil their responsibilities and help meet the aims set out in the statement of general policy.

6   What you cover and the amount of detail you record will reflect the level of risk, size, nature and complexity of the home. You do not need to repeat what is in another documents such as the infection control policy - a cross reference will suffice.

7   In successful policies, arrangements often include the following:

Monitoring
- Names of people (eg manager/competent person) nominated to carry out inspections, in conjunction with the safety representative, of the premises, equipment, systems of work and training needs.
- Intervals chosen for the inspection.
- Arrangements for internal reporting and investigation of accidents, near misses and cases of ill health; investigations should be aimed at finding immediate and underlying causes and the steps needed to prevent a reoccurrence.

- Where appropriate, periodic analysis of accident/ill-health records.
- Reporting of results of inspections and investigations to senior people within the organisation.

Training
- Identification of training needs of employees, including individual managers having direct responsibilities for health and safety.
- Provision of adequate health and safety training on recruitment and when risks to employees change, eg when they change job or use different equipment.

Supervision
- The need for adequate supervision of staff, particularly the young and new employees.

New equipment
- Arrangements for the assessment (from a health and safety viewpoint) of new equipment, eg new beds, hoists, building alterations.
- Least-hazardous options to be selected wherever possible.

Updates from suppliers
- Arrangements for seeing that health and safety bulletins from the Department of Health and other bodies are acted upon.

Reporting arrangements
- The reporting of injuries, dangerous occurrences and diseases to the appropriate enforcing authority.

Contractors and visitors
- Control of contractors including, for example, precontract meetings to discuss the health and safety implications of work contracted out and proposals for monitoring the health and safety performance during the work.
- Measures to identify and record asbestos in the fabric of the building and to prevent inadvertent exposure.
- The arrangements for the safety of visitors, eg in case of fire, potential violence etc.

Occupational health arrangements
- The provision of first-aid training, equipment and facilities.
- Health surveillance if appropriate.

Housekeeping
- Provision of orderly layout and defined passageways.
- Frequency of cleaning and waste removal.
- Clearing of spillages.

Safe systems of work
- The safe systems of work for particular operations, eg electrical and mechanical isolation and lock-off procedures during plant maintenance.

Planned maintenance
- Maintenance of the workplace, equipment, lifts, electrical apparatus etc in safe and efficient working order.

Exposure to substances
- The control of exposure to substances hazardous to health (COSHH). Arrangements for identifying the harmful substances, obtaining the appropriate data sheets from suppliers, assessing and controlling the risks.

Moving and handling
- Arrangements for meeting the Manual Operations Regulations 1992.

Transport and storage
- The organisation of traffic routes, training of those members of staff who drive minibuses etc.
- The arrangements for the safe stacking of materials.

Consultation

8   Most employers with effective safety policies find that consultation with employees is crucial if the proposals in the safety policy are to be realistic, acceptable and effective. Employers have to consult appointed safety representatives on issues specified in regulation 4A(1) of the Safety Representatives and Safety Committees Regulations 1977[3] as amended.

Publishing the health and safety policy

9   How you bring the policy to the notice of your employees will normally be determined the size and structure of your company. Access to the complete policy should be available to all employees and its existence brought to their attention.

10   It is vital that the policy is checked to see if what is said should be done is done. Without this the policy is just an empty gesture. It is important that when managers manage a health and safety performance they see not only what has been achieved but what has gone wrong or not been accomplished, not in order to lay blame, but to understand and remedy the chain of events that led to the failure.

Appendix 5 Working time

1   The Working Time Regulations 1998 set out maximum hours that workers should work. A worker is someone who undertakes work or a service for another party or employer. This includes the majority of agency workers and freelancers. Young persons are those between school leaving age and 18. The Regulations do not apply to the generally self-employed or volunteers unless there is a contract for a regular service.

2   Working time is defined as when someone is working at their employer's disposal and carrying out their activity or duties. This includes travelling, which is part of the job, working lunches, on-call time at worker's place of work and job-related training.

3   Working time does not include travelling between home and work, lunch breaks, evening classes or day release courses where they are not job related, or on-call time when the worker is free to pursue leisure activities. The working time limits do not apply to workers who can decide when they will work and how long they work.

4   Workers cannot be forced to work for more than 48 hours per week on an average. Average weekly time is normally calculated over 17 weeks. This period can be longer in certain situations, or workers and employers can agree to extend it.

5   Workers can agree to work longer than 48 hours a week. An agreement must be in writing and signed by the worker. It does not need to be renewed and employers only need to keep a record of workers who have signed an opt-out. Workers can cancel the opt-out agreement whenever they want, although they must give the employer at least seven days notice or longer (up to three months) if this has been agreed.

6   Employers cannot force workers to sign an opt-out. Workers cannot be fairly dismissed or subjected to detriment for refusing to sign an opt-out.

Working at night

7   A night worker is somebody who works at least three hours at night on a regular basis. Night time is the period between 11 pm and 6 am, although workers and employers may agree to vary this. Night workers should not work more than eight hours a day on average: this does not include overtime except regular overtime. If night workers work less than 48 hours a week, they are not exceeding this limit and so no further action is required.

8   Employers must offer night workers a free health assessment before they start working nights and thereafter on a regular basis while working nights. Workers do not have to take the opportunity to have a health assessment but it must be offered by the employer. Employers will need to keep a record of when and to whom the offer was made.

9   A health assessment is normally made up of two parts: a questionnaire and then a medical examination if there are doubts about the worker's fitness for night work. You may choose not to offer a questionnaire but start with a medical examination although this may be more expensive. You should get help from a suitably qualified health professional when devising and assessing the questionnaire. This may be from a doctor or nurse who understands how night working might affect health.

10   If a worker suffers from problems which are caused or made worse by night work, the employer should, if possible, transfer them to day work. Special consideration should be given to young workers' suitability for night work, taking account of their physique, maturity and experience.

Rest

11   Workers are entitled to 11 hours uninterrupted rest between each working day. Young workers are entitled to a 12-hour break between each working day.

12   Workers are entitled to 24 hours consecutive rest per week, or one 48-hour period or two 24 hour-periods of rest in every two weeks. Young workers are entitled to 48 hours consecutive rest each week. Days off are in addition to paid annual leave.

Rest breaks

13   Workers are entitled to a break of at least 20 minutes if they work for more than six hours. Young workers are entitled to a rest break of at least 30 minutes if they work for more than four and a half hours. Rest breaks are not in addition to lunch breaks.

14   It is up to the employer and the workers to agree between them whether the breaks are paid. In many cases, this will already be determined by an existing contract.

15   Exceptions can be made to these rules in the case of care homes. For more information, please contact your local HSE office.

Paid annual leave

16   Every worker, whether part-time or full-time, is entitled to four weeks paid annual leave. Workers are entitled to paid leave after they have been employed for 13 weeks.

17   A week's leave should allow workers to be away from the work for a week. It should be the same amount of time as the working week, if a worker does a five-day week, they are entitled to 20 days' leave; if they do a three-day week, the entitlement is 12 days' leave. The leave entitlement is not additional to Bank Holidays. There is no statutory right to take Bank Holidays off.

18   Workers must give their employer notice that they want to take leave. Employers can set the times workers take their leave and may not pay their employees not to take their leave.

19   Employers must make sure that workers can take their leave but are not required to make sure workers take their leave.

20   If a worker's employment ends, they have a right to be paid for the leave term that they are due but have not taken.

21   HSE and the local authorities only have responsibility for enforcing the working time limits and provisions for night working. Rest and leave entitlements are enforced through employment tribunals. For more information on Working Time Regulations, please refer to the book *Your guide to the Working Time Regulations*[29] produced by the Department of Trade and Industry.

Acknowledgements

HSE gratefully acknowledges all those who have contributed to this guidance, especially:

M Burns, British Federation of Care Home Proprietors

H Daley, UNISON

P Lown, Borough of Poole

C Purcell, Independent Sector Adviser, RCN

M Robson of Robson Associates

R Strange, Forum for Nurses Working with Older People, RCN

F Ursell, Registered Nursing Home Association

E White, HSE

References

1   *Draft guide to fire precautions in existing residential care premises* Home Office/Scottish Office 1983. Available from the Fire Policy Unit, Room 603, Horseferry House, Dean Ryle Street, London SW1P 2AW

2   *Health and Safety at Work etc Act 1974* The Stationery Office ISBN 0 10 543774 3

3   *Safety Representatives and Safety Committee Regulations 1977* SI 1977/500 The Stationery Office 1977 ISBN 0 11 070500 9

4   *The Health and Safety (Consultation with Employees) Regulations 1996* SI 1996/1513 The Stationery Office 1996 ISBN 0 11 054839 6

5   *Health and safety law: What you should know* (Poster) HSE Books 1999 ISBN 0 7176 2493 5

6   *Health and safety law: What you should know* (Leaflet) HSE Books 1999 (single copy free or priced packs of 25 ISBN 0 7176 1702 5)

7   *Management of health and safety at work. Management of Health and Safety at Work Regulations 1999. Approved Code of Practice* L21 (Second edition) HSE Books 2000 ISBN 0 7176 2488 9

8   *Successful health and safety management* HSG65 (Second edition) HSE Books 1997 ISBN 0 7176 1276 7

9   *Managing health and safety: Five steps to success* Leaflet INDG275 HSE Books 1998

10   *Five steps to risk assessment* Leaflet INDG163(rev1) HSE Books 1998 (single copy free or priced packs of 10 ISBN 0 7176 1565 0)

11   *A guide to the Reporting of Injuries, Diseases and Dangerous Occurrences Regulations 1995* L73 (Second edition) HSE Books 1999 ISBN 0 7176 2431 5

12   *The Reporting of Injuries, Diseases and Dangerous Occurrences Regulations 1995: Guidance for employers in the healthcare sector* Health Services Information Sheet HSIS1 HSE Books 1998

13   *First aid at work. The Health and Safety (First Aid) Regulations 1981. Approved Code of Practice and guidance* L74 HSE Books 1997 ISBN 0 7176 1050 0

14   *General COSHH ACOP (Control of substances hazardous to health) and Carcinogens ACOP (Control of carcinogenic substances) and Biological agents ACOP (Control of biological agents). Control of Substances Hazardous to Health Regulations 1999. Approved Codes of Practice* L5 (Third edition) HSE Books 1999 ISBN 0 7176 1670 3

15   *Latex and you* Leaflet INDG320 HSE Books 2000 (single copy free or priced packs of 10 ISBN 0 7176 1777 7)

16   *Safe disposal of clinical waste* HSE Books (Second edition) 1999 ISBN 0 7176 2492 7

17   *Manual Handling Operations Regulations 1992. Guidance on Regulations* L23 (Second edition) HSE Books 1998 ISBN 0 7176 2415 3

18   *Safe use of lifting equipment. Lifting Operations and Lifting Equipment Regulations 1998. Approved Code of Practice and guidance* L113 HSE Books 1998 ISBN 0 7176 1628 2

19   *Violence and aggression to staff in health services: Guidance on assessment and management* HSE Books 1997 ISBN 0 7176 1466 2

20   *Tackling work-related stress: A manager's guide to improving and maintaining employee health and well-being* HSG218 HSE Books 2001 ISBN 0 7176 2050 6

21   *Tackling work-related stress: A guide for employees* INDG341 HSE Books 2001 (single copy free or priced packs of 20 ISBN 0 7176 2065 4)

22   *Legionnaires' disease. The control of legionella bacteria in water systems. Approved Code of Practice and guidance* L8 (Second edition) HSE Books 2001 ISBN 0 7176 1772 6

23   *'Safe' hot water and surface temperatures* NHS Estates Guidance Note: 1998 ISBN 0 11 321404 9

24   *Safety in the installation and use of gas systems and appliances. Gas Safety (Installation and Use) Regulations 1998. Approved Code of Practice and guidance* L56 (Second edition) HSE Books 1998 ISBN 0 7176 1635 5

25   *Memorandum of guidance on the Electricity at Work Regulations 1989. Guidance on Regulations* HSR25 HSE Books 1989 ISBN 0 7176 1602 9

26   *Electrical safety and you* Leaflet INDG231 HSE Books 1996 (single copy free or priced packs of 15 ISBN 0 7176 1207 4)

27   *Workplace health, safety and welfare. Workplace (Health, Safety and Welfare) Regulations 1992. Approved Code of Practice* L24 HSE Books 1992 ISBN 0 7176 0413 6

28   *Pesticides: Use them safely* Leaflet INDG257 HSE Books 1997

29   *Your guide to the Working Time Regulations* DTI March 2000 (Contact the DTI Publications Orderline: 0870 150 2500)

Further reading

Essentials of health and safety at work
(Second edition) HSE Books 1994 ISBN 0 7176 0716 X

Young people at work: A guide for employers HSG165
(Second edition) HSE Books 2000 ISBN 0 7176 1889 7

Be safe save money: The costs of accidents - A guide for small firms Leaflet INDG208 HSE Books 1995

Stating your business. Guidance on preparing a health and safety policy statement Leaflet INDG324
HSE Books 2000 (single copy free or priced packs of 5
ISBN 0 7176 1799 8)

First aid at work: Your questions answered Leaflet
INDG214 HSE Books 1997 (single copy free or priced
packs of 15 ISBN 0 7176 1074 8)

A step by step guide to COSHH assessment HSG97
HSE Books 1993 ISBN 0 7176 1446 8

COSHH a brief guide to the Regulations: What you need to know about the Control of Substances Hazardous to Health Regulations 1999 (COSHH)
Leaflet INDG136(rev1) HSE Books 1999 (single copy free or priced packs of 10 ISBN 0 7176 2444 7)

Guidance for Clinical Healthcare Workers: Protection against infection with HIV and Hepatitis Viruses - Recommendations of the expert advisory group on AIDS Department of Health ISBN 0 11 321249 6

Getting to grips with manual handling: A short guide for employers Leaflet INDG143(rev1) HSE Books 2000
(single copy free or priced packs of 15
ISBN 0 7176 1754 8)

Manual handling in the health services (Second edition) HSE Books 1998 ISBN 0 7176 1248 1

Preventing violence to staff HSE/Tavistock Institute of Human Relations HSE Books 1988 ISBN 0 11 885467 4

Controlling legionella in nursing and residential care homes Leaflet INDG253 HSE Books 1997

Asbestos essentials task manual: Task guidance sheets for the building maintenance and allied trades
HSG210 HSE Books 2001 ISBN 0 7176 1887 0

Working with asbestos in buildings Leaflet INDG289
HSE Books 1999 (single copy free or priced packs of
10 ISBN 0 7176 1697 5)

Managing asbestos in workplace buildings Leaflet
INDG223(rev1) HSE Books 1996 (single copy free or
priced packs of 10 ISBN 0 7176 1179 5)

Preventing slips, trips and falls at work Leaflet
INDG225 HSE Books 1996 (single copy free or priced
packs of 15 ISBN 0 7176 1183 3)

The Lifts Regulations 1997 The Stationery Office 1997
ISBN 0 11 064274 0

Safe use of lifting equipment. Lifting Operations and Lifting Equipment Regulations 1998. Approved Code of Practice and guidance L113 HSE Books 1998
ISBN 0 7176 1628 2

Passive smoking at work Leaflet INDG63(rev1) HSE
Books 1992 (single copy free or priced packs of 10
ISBN 0 7176 0882 4)

Health and safety in kitchens and food preparation areas HSG55 HSE Books 1990 ISBN 0 7176 0492 6

Reporting incidents of exposure to pesticides and veterinary medicines Leaflet INDG141(rev1)
HSE Books 1999

A short guide to the Working Time Regulations August
2000 DTI leaflet (Contact the DTI Publications
Orderline: 0870 150 2500)

VDUs: An easy guide to the regulations HSG90 HSE
Books 1994 ISBN 0 7176 0735 6

Standards

ISO 9386 *Power-operated platforms for persons with impaired mobility - Rules for safety, dimensions and functional operation. Part 1: Vertical lifting platforms. Part 2: Powered stair lifts for seated, standing and wheelchair users moving in an inclined plane*

BS EN 81 *Safety rules for the construction and installation of lifts. Part 1: Electric lifts.
Part 2: Hydraulic lifts*

BS EN 60309: *Plugs, socket outlets and couplers for industrial purposes*

BS EN 61008: *Specification for residual current-operated circuit-breakers without integral overcurrent protection for household and similar uses (RCCBS).* Part 1: *General rules*

BS 1363: 1984 *Specification for 13A fused plugs and switched and unswitched electrical outlets*

BS 4293: 1983 *Specification for residual current-operated circuit-breakers*

BS 5776: 1996 *Specification for powered stair lifts*

BS 5900: 1999 *Specification for powered domestic lifts with partially enclosed cars and no lift well enclosures*

BS 6262: 1982 *Code of practice for glazing in buildings*

BS 6440: 1999 *Powered lifting platforms for use by disabled persons - Code of practice*

BS 6642: 1985 *Specification for disposable plastics refuse sacks made from polyethylene*

BS 7071: 1992 *Specification for portable residual current devices*

BS 7320: 1990 *Specification for sharps containers*

BS 7671: 1992 *Requirements for electrical installations. IEE Wiring Regulations (Sixteenth edition)*

While every effort has been made to ensure the accuracy of the references listed in this publication, their future availability cannot be guaranteed.

HSE priced and free publications are available by mail order from HSE Books, PO Box 1999, Sudbury, Suffolk CO10 2WA Tel: 01787 881165 Fax: 01787 313995 Website: www.hsebooks.co.uk (HSE priced publications are also available from bookshops.)

British Standards are available from BSI Customer Services, 389 Chiswick High Road, London W4 4AL Tel: 020 8996 9001 Fax: 020 8996 7001 Website: www.bsi-global.com

The Stationery Office (formerly HMSO) publications are available from The Publications Centre, PO Box 276, London SW8 5DT Tel: 0870 600 5522 Fax: 0870 600 5533 Website: www.clicktso.com (They are also available from bookshops.)

Further information

Medical Devices Agency
Hannibal House
Elephant and Castle
London SE1 6TQ
Tel: 020 7972 8000
Email: mail@medical-devices.gov.uk

Printed and published by the Health and Safety Executive
C200   12/01